The

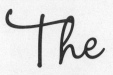

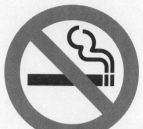

HOW TO QUIT
SMOKING
AND NOT GAIN
WEIGHT
COOKBOOK

Also by Mary Donkersloot, R.D.

The Simply Gourmet Diabetes Cookbook

The

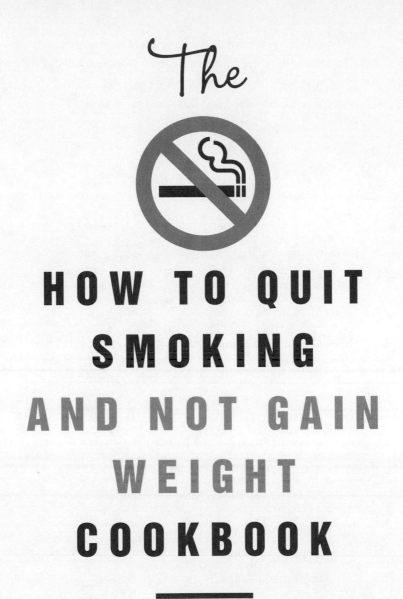

HOW TO QUIT
SMOKING
AND NOT GAIN
WEIGHT
COOKBOOK

MARY DONKERSLOOT, R.D., AND LINDA HYDER FERRY, M.D., M.P.H.

THREE RIVERS PRESS
NEW YORK

This book is dedicated to all the smokers who gave up on a smoke-free future because they were afraid of gaining weight. We hope someone gives them a copy of this book and says, "It's dedicated to *you*!"

Copyright © 1999 by Mary Donkersloot and Linda Hyder Ferry

Published by Three Rivers Press, 201 East 50th Street, New York, New York 10022. Member of the Crown Publishing Group.

Random House, Inc. New York, Toronto, London, Sydney, Auckland
www.randomhouse.com

THREE RIVERS PRESS is a registered trademark of Random House, Inc.

Printed in the United States of America

Design by Elizabeth van Itallie

Library of Congress Cataloging-in-Publication Data
Donkersloot, Mary
The how to quit smoking and not gain weight cookbook / by Mary
Donkersloot and Linda Hyder Ferry.
1. Cigarette smokers—Diet therapy Recipes.   2. Smoking—
Prevention.   I. Hyder Ferry, Linda.   II. Title.
RC567.D66   1999
616.86'50654—dc21   99-25276
                                                        CIP

ISBN 0-609-80363-8

10 9 8 7 6 5 4 3 2 1

FIRST EDITION

Acknowledgments

Our thanks begin with a salute to Brigit Binns and Peter Kleiner, who offered their wisdom, creative input, and assistance with manuscript preparation.

Every book has a lineup of "behind the scenes heroes" that take an idea and transform it into a tangible reality. We want every one of you to know how grateful we are for your meaningful contribution. The suggestion that put the whole idea in motion originated from Ed Weinstock. Next are our agents, Maureen and Eric Lasher, who encouraged us to move ahead and launch our project. Gary Stanhiser skillfully worked out the joint agreement that brought the two authors together. Katie Workman, our editor, was enthusiastic about this book from the beginning and skillfully guided it through the editing and rewriting phase. Julia Coblentz and the entire crew at Clarkson N. Potter have shown calm dedication and commitment in turning our manuscript into a readable book. Wendy Schuman gave her great talents in promotion and public relations to let the world know the valuable information in this book.

Our gratitude to Sara Jaye, whose enthusiastic recipe testing and boundless culinary creativity made this a fun and delicious project.

Steve Proffitt deserves special praise for his love and assistance on a daily basis. To Miriam Perec, a thank you for constant support and vital input.

For expert opinion on nicotine and food cravings, we turned to Dr. Neil Grunberg and Elizabeth Somer, M.A., R.D. The tried and true tips from the trenches of exercise physiology came from Bob Antonacci, M.S., Susan Block, M.S., and Leslie Goetzman, M.S.

Many colleagues offered support, encouragement, expertise, and thoughtful insight, not to mention speedy manuscript reading: Lisa Carlson, M.S., R.D.; Susan Dopart, M.S., R.D.; Barbara Chizmas; Dona Constantine, B.A., R.N.; Rani Williams; Linda Grissino Evans, M.D., M.P.H.; Judith E. Hyder, M.A., R.N., and David Ross Ferry, M.D.; Robert Guy Hyder, Ph.D.; Janet Lepke, R.D., C.D.E., L.D.N.; Anthony Reading, Ph.D.; and Barbara Rolls, Ph.D.

Thousands of smokers donated their time to medical research in the quest for answers about why people gain weight after giving up tobacco. We trust that the real-world wisdom their insight and struggles provide is inspirational to all who read this book.

Contents

FOREWORD BY C. EVERETT KOOP, M.D. xi

INTRODUCTION 1

Part One

CHAPTER 1 The Link Between Smoking and Weight Change 9

CHAPTER 2 You Can Do It! 16

CHAPTER 3 Coping with Cravings After Smoking Cessation 38

CHAPTER 4 Ten Steps: Eating for Health 50

CHAPTER 5 The Personal Nutrition Management Plan with Menu Plans 66

CHAPTER 6 Motivation: Change Your Thoughts, Change Your Behavior ...98

CHAPTER 7 Exercise Is Key 108

CHAPTER 8 Smart Snacking That Satisfies 116

CHAPTER 9 Dining Out Tips 130

Part Two

CHAPTER 10 A New Way of Cooking 145

CHAPTER 11 Breakfast and Brunch........................151

CHAPTER 12 Appetizers 166

CHAPTER 13 Soups 171

CHAPTER 14 Salads 183

CHAPTER 15 Main Courses: Fish, Chicken, Lean Meats 201

CHAPTER 16 Pasta and Pizza 228

CHAPTER 17 Sandwiches and Wraps 238

CHAPTER 18 Side Dishes 247

CHAPTER 19 Desserts 261

APPENDIX 276

How to Calculate Your Calorie Need 276

Nutritional Value Counter 277

Stop-Smoking Resources 293

Notes 299

Index 301

Foreword

By C. Everett Koop, M.D.

Two important problems that have increased in the American lifestyle in this century are tobacco use and behaviors leading to obesity. The first is largely a result of promotion and marketing by the tobacco industry. The second is the natural outcome of sedentary lifestyles and an abundance of refined and high-fat "convenience foods."

The fear of gaining weight after quitting tobacco use is a significant barrier that prevents hundreds of thousands of smokers from even attempting to quit. This is why Linda Hyder Ferry, M.D., M.P.H., and Mary Donkersloot, R.D., teamed up to bring their experience and expertise from the fields of medicine and nutrition to produce a reliable guide for smokers who want the best advice on quitting smoking without the consequence of significant weight gain.

While it is common knowledge that ex-smokers often gain weight shortly after quitting, there has not been an in-depth explanation to date that is helpful to smokers. The authors have included practical tips and recipes for a healthy and delicious way to celebrate the return of a normal appetite and an enhanced sense of smell and taste after quitting smoking, without overindulging and fearing the tally on the bathroom scales. The emerging science of neurochemistry allows us to understand how nicotine is involved in the regulation of appetite and pleasure centers in the brain. New medications that address these processes coupled with sensible eating patterns can make the transition to a smoke-free future much easier. Armed with this information smokers can confidently create a smoke-free lifestyle that was previously an unrealistic hope.

The authors point out clearly that just reacting to the weight gain by "starving" yourself, using restrictive dieting cycles or being overwhelmed with cravings and urges for food, is counterproductive. This usually leads to unwanted weight gain or relapse back to smoking when the pounds start piling on.

While the fear of weight gain is "larger than life," most ex-smokers only gain an average of 4.5 pounds. In fact, some people gain no weight at all, and less than 3 percent gain over 20 pounds. After 10 years, the average weight of ex-smokers increased to that of never-smokers, not heavier! The real consequences of continuing to smoke versus gaining less than 10 pounds are far more serious. In one to two years after quitting, most ex-smokers are back to normal weight.

As we move into the twenty-first-century, American smokers need to turn to their health-care professionals for a sensible approach to quitting tobacco using all the tools now available. Three disciplines include behavioral counseling to extinguish the rituals of tobacco use, the nutritional advice to adopt healthy eating habits—not new food addictions, and the medical support to treat nicotine withdrawal by stabilizing the neurochemistry that drives addictions.

We are capable of much higher success rates than we had even a decade ago thanks to the clearer understanding of the way the brain reacts to nicotine. This is the best time in history to quit smoking.

The majority (70 percent) of smokers say they want to quit smoking, but the strength of the nicotine addiction and the barriers that impair their progress keep them trapped in the belief that they don't have the "willpower" or ability to succeed. The gamble is so deadly and the stakes are so high (one out of three smokers will die prematurely of a tobacco-related disease) that we can't sit back and watch smokers slowly kill themselves for fear of gaining weight. Every smoker needs to hear this message loud and clear—

1. There is no better time than now to quit.
2. Don't let anything stand in your way. Learn how to quit smoking without developing a compensating addiction like food.
3. Get professional medical help to help you overcome the reasons you fear quitting smoking.
4. Move out of that smoke-filled cloud and into the smoke-free future you have hoped for.

If all smokers who have hesitated in the past to quit smoking for fear of weight gain took the advice offered in this book, we would see the death rates fall over the next decade from tobacco-related diseases. Let's work together to achieve this goal.

Introduction

FACING OUR FEARS AND ADDICTIONS

In 1995, an estimated 47 million adults in the United States identified themselves as smokers.[1] There is no doubt that most—if not all—of these people know the health risks of smoking. Yet 22 percent of women and 27 percent of men continue to smoke. Of the 70 percent of smokers who say they want to quit each year, only 1 to 2 percent quit permanently.

The high failure rate for those who attempt to stop smoking is alarming. Clearly scare tactics don't work. But are smokers just lacking in willpower, incapable of following through on their convictions? Although there are many explanations for this failure rate, one excuse is common: "I gained twenty pounds the last time I tried to quit smoking, and I just can't afford to do that again."

This book is for people who want to stop smoking but are afraid of gaining weight and for those who have successfully stopped smoking and have gained unwanted pounds as a result.

Beyond the fear of gaining weight, recognize that a more insidious force is at work here, one that sabotages smokers' efforts on several different levels. Perhaps you've heard the irritating claim of ex-smokers who "just decided to stop smoking, and then did it." This is by far the rarity. But if you view smoking as a physical addiction, and acknowledge that quitting will take some effort to accomplish successfully (i.e., without gaining weight or alienating those near and dear to you), then you are much more likely to win the battle.

"QUITTING IS EASY, I'VE DONE IT A HUNDRED TIMES. . . ."

There is no shortage of information on the negative health aspects of smoking. Every year, more studies are published detailing the frightening statistics on heart disease, lung cancer, emphysema, and the risks of exposure to second-hand smoke. Most smokers, however, believe that these documented hazards of smoking will not touch them personally, and many honestly believe they can quit any time they really want to. That is, until they try and fail.

THE DECISION TO QUIT

The decision to quit smoking is an important one, affecting you, your family, and even the people you work with. It's a decision that will lead to all kinds of benefits, not the least of which is an increased life span and better overall health. The positive effects of quitting smoking are so compelling that non-smokers have trouble understanding why anyone still smokes.

A serious obstacle for many smokers is that weight gain is a frequent side effect, and one with very negative implications. In the short-term view, weight gain can seem more of an evil than continuing to smoke. In other words, people would rather keep smoking, risking their lives and the lives of those around them on a daily basis, than gain weight. But it doesn't have to be that way, and that's why you picked up this book. To follow through on the decision to quit smoking, it is helpful to understand why people smoke in the first place.

ADDICTIVE THINKING

Let's face it: People smoke because they enjoy smoking. Just as cocaine addicts like to use cocaine, and alcoholics like to drink, because both drugs make them feel happy, or better about life, smokers use cigarettes because they stimulate the brain chemistry and provide pleasurable sensations. (See page 20 for a more detailed explanation.) These are familiar sentiments from people involved in addictive behaviors. Addicts are unable to see the consequences of their choices, and this is the very nature of addictive thinking. The drug makes the addict do anything to keep acquiring the feeling provided by the drug, regardless of the emotional, financial, and occupational costs, or the effects on personal relationships. Smokers learn to live in denial of the seriousness of their addiction and its consequences because in the short term, smoking is pleasurable. An addictive personality often becomes addicted to more than one substance. Making sure that food is not the next addiction is an important key in the process of quitting smoking without gaining weight.

CONQUERING THE FEAR OF QUITTING

Barriers to quitting are a reality; otherwise, we would see a much higher success rate for all the smokers who try to stop every year. Fear of failure, fear of weight gain, fear of mood swings—these are all factors that justifiably concern potential ex-smokers. Peer support is another important issue—if a smoker believes he does not have enough support from friends and family, then he will have more difficulty overcoming the urge to smoke.

Mood swings—a common cause for failure—should not be discounted as unimportant. Anxiety, depression, restlessness, irritability, anger, difficulty in concentrating, and difficulty in sleeping are realities for the quitting smoker. Patients at a stop-smoking clinic will often say: "I couldn't stand myself, and worse, no one else could stand me either—I was so irritable, frustrated, even angry. It seemed like these feelings would go on forever, so I just gave up." Another quitter confided, "My biggest concern is how I reacted at work. I just can't afford to be so irritable with my customers, disagreeable to my employees, and unable to concentrate. I've never been able to stay off cigarettes for a whole week without feeling overwhelmed by these withdrawal symptoms." These are serious concerns, but shouldn't intimidate prospective ex-smokers. Acknowledging and confronting these fears in advance, and understanding that mood swings are part of the experience, will increase the likelihood that the quitting attempt succeeds.

STACK THE CARDS IN YOUR FAVOR: HOW TO USE THIS BOOK

You do not have to accept the inevitability of permanent or even short-term weight gain. There *is* something you can do, and it starts with being prepared by understanding the reasons why so many people gain weight after they quit smoking. If you read and use this book in a methodical way, you'll have everything at hand to successfully adapt to a smoke-free lifestyle. Then, of course, you must follow through with your commitments; otherwise, all your time and effort will be wasted.

In Chapter 1, you'll learn about the relationship between smoking and weight changes. What you discover may surprise and even frighten you, because there is a direct cause and effect between the two. Once you understand the relationship, however, you'll be well-armed against the negative effects that could result when you take a very positive step in your life and quit smoking.

In Chapter 2, find out how smoking and nicotine affect your brain and body, and how much you have to gain by quitting. Take a quiz to identify your motivation for smoking, and then learn how to replace it with an activity that's beneficial to your well-being. Define the "type" of smoker you are, and learn how to replace what you get from tobacco with healthier pursuits. You'll also learn how to identify the symptoms of nicotine withdrawal, and how today's effective drugs can help allay those symptoms and keep you on target.

Food cravings are a difficult hurdle for many, and are typically experienced in the first two to six weeks after quitting. In Chapter 3, find out why quitting smokers experience these cravings, and why certain foods can become almost irresistible. You'll learn the biological basis for food cravings, and how eating just a small amount of the right food can satisfy them—there's no need to binge.

In Chapter 4, you'll find detailed guidelines that will get you nutritionally on track at this critical time in your life. Here, you'll find a helpful personal nutrition plan, a 10-step plan for those who would like to quit smoking, and those who have already quit. You'll learn why popular diets often don't work in the long run, and how taking a new, more flexible approach to food vastly increases your chances of success over a strict diet.

Chapter 5 is composed of the Personal Nutrition Management Plan. This is the first step for quitters who have successfully remained off nicotine for 12 weeks or more. If you quit smoking some time ago (six months ago, for example) and you are still carrying more weight than you are comfortable with, then this chapter is for you. At this point, you are beyond the greatest danger of relapsing. Included are three weeks of menu plans to help you make healthy food choices, incorporating all your favorite foods without feeling deprived.

Chapters 6, 7, and 8 address the important subjects of good exercise, smart snacking, and, of course, motivation in terms of quitting smoking and maintaining your weight. Learn how to live with a few mistakes and emphasize positive accomplishments to keep your program squarely on target. Remember, this is the rest of your life that's at stake. Don't sabotage your efforts with self-defeating thoughts.

Finally, 100 simple and delicious recipes will help you bring the Personal Nutrition Management Plan into your life and your home. These recipes, made with easily accessible ingredients, are dishes that your friends and family can enjoy right along with you. You'll never feel deprived when feasting on Old-Fashioned Beef Stew, Chicken Jambalaya, and Crunchy Oatmeal Chocolate Chip Cookies. This section also includes many helpful tips on healthy eating: Learn how to cut back on saturated fat by using olive oil or canola oil instead of butter, and how to use egg whites as a substitute for whole eggs, when possible. Discover how to emphasize vegetables and fruits in every meal as well.

Working through the chapters of this book and following the personalized, step-by-step plan will give you an understanding of the pitfalls that await as you attempt this very important step for your future well-being. More important, you'll be able to apply this information and advice to your own life. Making a change for the better—while avoiding the pitfalls—will fill you with a satisfied feeling of intense pride and accomplishment. You may even lose a few pounds. Congratulations! You're on the way to a healthier, fitter, and happier you.

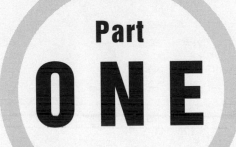

Part

ONE

CHAPTER 1
The Link Between
Smoking and
Weight Change

In the minds of many people, smoking cessation is connected with weight gain, and for good reason. The medical and nutrition community has a clear understanding of why many ex-smokers gain weight for a period just after they quit. But these reasons have not been fully explained to the smoking public. Although there are psychological factors to weight gain, many are physical, and involve the effects of nicotine on the brain and the changes that occur when nicotine is discontinued. A monumental and powerful struggle takes place during the transition from a nicotine-dependent brain to a nicotine-free brain.

People gain weight when they quit smoking for several reasons:
- Smokers are used to a "hand-to-mouth" habit and often replace that habit with eating.
- Nicotine withdrawal symptoms can stimulate a craving for food.
- When the sense of smell returns after being paralyzed by smoking, the wonderful smell and taste of food can be extremely tempting and lead to overeating.
- Smoking speeds the metabolism so fat burns faster. Quitting slows the metabolism, and exercise must be increased to compensate.

Understanding and anticipating these consequences will help ex-smokers and future ex-smokers attain the positive health benefits of stopping smoking without gaining weight.

IS WEIGHT GAIN AN UNAVOIDABLE SIDE EFFECT?

Many prospective quitters face the fear of weight gain: "The last time I tried to quit smoking, I gained a lot of weight. . . . I can't face doing that again." It's a frequent complaint, but there's another interesting, and disturbing, statistic: An estimated 40 percent of female smokers say they use nicotine as a means of managing their weight. A study just published, however, found that smoking does not prevent normal weight gain for people under the age of 30,[1] based on the results of following nearly 4,000 young adults between the ages of 18 and 30 for seven years. Yet despite the evidence that young smokers put on weight just as readily as nonsmokers, one in four continue to smoke because of the fear of weight gain. In other words, the prospect of looking in a mirror today scares them more than the idea of looking at an X ray of their lungs in 20 years.

The consequence of weight gain has become a widely accepted side effect of smoking cessation, and the reason for many relapses. But most people don't really understand why post-cessation weight gain occurs, much less know how to stop themselves from joining the statistics. If the fear of weight gain has prevented you from making an attempt to quit, consider what happens when nicotine stops circulating in the brain to help put the problem in perspective.

Cause and Effect: Smoking and Weight Changes

Let's set the record straight. Weight gain after quitting is not inevitable!

The average amount of weight gained by quitting smokers is 4.5 pounds. This means that some people gain no weight, many people gain from 5 to 8 pounds, and a few people (less than 3 percent) gain over 20 pounds. But after 10 years, ex-smokers have been found to weigh the same as those who never smoked. So the physiological effects that cause weight gain are only temporary, and can be avoided altogether with a little planning.

On average, smokers weigh less than nonsmokers. The reasons for this are not complicated.

> **1.** Smoking dulls the appetite. Nicotine is a potent appetite suppressant, and many people who have smoked since their teens have never experienced a fully active and healthy adult appetite.

2. Smoking is toxic to the sense of smell. Tobacco smoke paralyzes the olfactory nerve in the nose, which controls the sense of smell.

3. Smoking speeds up the body's metabolism, causing fat and calories to burn off at a faster rate.

4. Smoking alters the normal distribution of body fat because the body's mechanism for producing and using energy is stimulated by nicotine. Weight accumulates at the waist instead of the hips as it would normally in a nonsmoker. This puts the smoker at a higher risk for heart disease.

When a smoker gives up nicotine, there is substantial change in all of the above mechanisms. The trick is to look at each one in a positive light.

1. Celebrate the return of a normal healthy adult appetite; it's a wonderful thing to enjoy. Just be sure you control it—don't let it control you!

2. An improved sense of smell—which for most people returns after one or two weeks of avoiding tobacco smoke—will enhance the taste and smell of food. Food is one of a healthy adult's most enjoyable pleasures. Gradually becoming aware of the subtle aromas of food will be a revelation, because food may smell and taste better than you ever expected. But that's no reason to eat larger than necessary portions!

3. A normal metabolism is healthier for the body and much more predictable. Learn to live with the metabolism you were born with.

4. Carrying weight on your hips instead of your waist will decrease your risk for heart disease.

In the excitement of returning to a normal body chemistry and normal enjoyment of food, watch out for these pitfalls:

1. Don't increase your overall food intake as a means of rewarding yourself. Just enjoy smaller quantities by savoring not overindulging your food.

2. Be careful of the side effects of nicotine cravings, which many quitters experience. Studies indicate that the craving for nicotine may be related to several chemicals in the brain that satisfy hunger and the desire for sugar. The result can be a craving for certain types of food, often high-fat and/or high-carbohydrate. The reasons for this are explored more fully in Chapter 3.

3. Smokers are accustomed to having "rituals" to perform with their hands—sometimes smokers light up out of nervousness just to keep their hands busy. Be careful not to substitute snacking on empty calories for smoking, which can add anywhere from 300 to 800 extra calories per day to your usual intake.

4. Smoking speeds up the body's metabolism, and quitting causes the metabolism to return to its normal, slower speed. Even if the new ex-smoker's calorie intake remains the same, the slower metabolism means that the body has no choice but to store the excess, unused calories or energy as fat. (Some experts claim that quitting nicotine adds another 200 calories to the system each day.) There is only one way to tip this equation in your favor: Use more energy—i.e., exercise. Even a moderate increase in the amount of exercise you do will stabilize the drop in metabolism and prevent normal calorie intake from being stored as fat.

UNDERSTANDING YOUR RELATIONSHIP WITH FOOD

Aside from smoking, you may have other habits that can cause problems with weight gain. It is helpful to identify those tendencies before they become a problem.

Do you use food to cope with feelings of depression, loneliness, anger, boredom, or frustration? Perhaps you respond too strongly to food cues like advertising, and the influence of those around you who may have less incentive to manage their calorie intake.

The following quiz will help you identify some of the behaviors that can put you at risk for weight gain after quitting smoking.

1. Do you eat sweets in an amount of 300 calories or more per serving, four times a week or more?

2. Do you regularly snack on chips, nuts, nachos, French fries, cookies, pastries, and other starchy foods, without paying attention to portion size?

3. Do you use large portions of margarine, butter, salad dressing, sour cream, and/or cheese on breads, salads, and other foods?

4. When cooking, do you add more than one teaspoon of oil to the pan per serving?

5. Do you regularly eat the skin on chicken, or the fat on beef?

6. Do you eat "typical" fast foods (not healthy fast foods) or fried foods more than once per week?

7. Do you regularly eat snacks like full-fat ice cream and other desserts?

8. Do you overeat healthy carbohydrate foods such as fruit, bagels, or pasta—rationalizing that they are good for you simply because they are fat-free? (Remember that excess calories, not just excess fat, can cause weight gain.)

9. Do you often eat when you're bored, depressed, angry, or happy—even if you are not hungry?

10. Do you often eat "unconsciously" while at the movies, watching television, or at a restaurant without responding to whether you are hungry or full?

If you answered "yes" to three or more of the above questions, you may be susceptible to weight gain after you stop smoking, not just due to the effects of nicotine withdrawal but also to your established eating habits.

WOMEN AT RISK

Women are often more concerned than men about weight gain after quitting smoking. Up to 55 percent of women say they have little or no confidence that they can control their weight if and when they quit smoking.

Unfortunately, cultural influences make women feel it is more acceptable to smoke than to carry a few extra pounds. But the excess pounds that often accompany cessation of smoking can be prevented. You may have already quit smoking before you bought this book and gained more weight than you had anticipated. Be reassured that once the body is truly free of the debilitating nicotine addiction, it will return to a natural, healthy weight within one to two years. If you are concerned about a recent weight gain after quitting, remember that all the health benefits enjoyed during the smoke-free stage will more than overshadow the temporary period of weighing a few pounds more.

KEEPING PERSPECTIVE: DON'T PANIC AT A FEW EXTRA POUNDS

The prospect of weight gain may discourage one in four smokers from even making the attempt to quit. This applies especially to smokers who are aware that they use tobacco to suppress a normal appetite and control their weight. But the direct health effects of a minor weight gain are trivial in comparison to the negative effects of continuing to smoke. By following the Personal Nutrition Management Plan detailed in this book, anyone should be able to avoid unnecessary weight gain after quitting smoking. The Personal Nutrition Management Plan is a healthy alternative that will allow you to live smoke-free without gaining weight. The key is maintaining a simple balancing act between the food you eat and the exercise you get. That's not to say it's easy; avoiding weight gain after quitting smoking takes hard work. Most people would agree that the rewards, which include a healthier lifestyle, an increased enjoyment of food, a wonderfully enhanced sense of smell, and, last but certainly not least, an increased life expectancy and quality of life are worth the effort. Don't you agree?

If you have struggled with the fear of gaining weight as an excuse for why you haven't stopped smoking, then this book can help. But if you are seriously concerned about your eating habits, consider these possible options:

1. Talk to a dietitian or health-care professional about your plan to quit smoking. Discuss your concerns about behaviors that predispose you to weight gain.

2. Consider using medications to control nicotine withdrawal symptoms, in consultation with your physician. Some medications have been shown to produce less weight gain after quitting than an effort without medication (more about these medications in Chapter 2).

3. Deal with the few extra pounds that may accrue after your addiction is under better control, perhaps after three months or so.

4. Most important of all, always remind yourself of the benefits you will gain by quitting. Focus on the positive!

EXCEPTIONS TO THE RULE

There are some individuals who shouldn't consider even temporary weight gain as acceptable. If you are diabetic, are already 40 percent above your ideal body weight, suffer from coronary heart disease, or have high blood pressure or high blood cholesterol levels, it would be unwise to allow a gain of even 15 to 20 pounds. Such people should consult a nutritionist or health-care professional *before* embarking on a quitting plan, still in conjunction with the Personal Nutritional Management Plan. Overweight smokers, especially, should read Chapter 3 and start a program of healthy nutrition and regular exercise to control their weight prior to quitting. Everyone benefits from increased exercise, but for these groups exercise is crucial to avoid potential weight gain.

CHAPTER 2
You Can Do It!

Fear of gaining weight is probably an important issue for you, and that's why you picked up this book. But so is your deep desire to eliminate tobacco from your life. You've decided that the pleasure gained from smoking simply doesn't justify the completely avoidable health consequences of nicotine addiction. For most people, however, quitting isn't just a matter of snapping your fingers and saying "I don't smoke anymore." This chapter is designed for the smoker who has failed before or is afraid of failure. You need not be a failure—if you are ready and determined to prepare for life without nicotine. We've covered several positive aspects of quitting, but there are obviously negative consequences as well. That's not an excuse not to quit, it's just a "heads up" to make sure you understand all the factors involved in a successful quit attempt.

Learning how to balance the positive and negative consequences of quitting can help you achieve the goal of living smoke-free permanently. Fortunately, the negative consequences are few and temporary. For instance, mood swings due to changes in the brain's chemistry may cause temporary disturbances in relationships with friends, family, and coworkers. You may become less likable for a little while. And you may find that your fear of gaining weight is blown all out of proportion. These factors can all be anticipated and managed, though probably not completely avoided. Your body has been on a powerful, addictive drug—getting off it will not be a cakewalk. This book can provide you with the tools, information, and confidence to make this your last quit attempt, with a bonus of a new and healthier lifestyle.

WHAT'S YOUR MOTIVATION FOR SMOKING? FOR QUITTING?

The chart on page 18 should help you identify the key reasons why you smoke so you can plan a successful quit attempt. Be honest in answering the questions. If you don't, the only person who'll lose out is you.

The Choice Is Yours

On the left side of the form on the next page, write all your reasons for wanting to quit in order of importance. Reasons may be health-related, financial, social, occupational, or family concerns about passive smoke exposure. Below each reason in the Result space, write what you will gain. For instance, Reason: I want to break free of the addictive cycle that tells me I must smoke in order to feel normal. Result: I will regain my self-respect since I will no longer be an addict.

Now on the right side of the form, write all the reasons for NOT wanting to quit, again in order of importance, and then fill in the result. For instance, Reason: Smoking when I get upset or nervous is so calming. Result: I will always be dependent on nicotine to help me handle the stress in my life.

As you prepare to quit, put this list in a place where you will see it several times a day so you can consider the results of your choices and actions. When you feel the need to smoke, read through your "Reasons" list before you reach for the cigarettes. Add more reasons to quit and anticipated results as the days go by, and let the impact sink in. Watch your resolve build and strengthen over several days as you clarify your values about smoking.

A FEW GOOD REASONS TO QUIT

You can't escape from the scary statistics on cigarette smoking, because they're serious enough to be a constant in everyone's life—smoker or not—at the end of the twentieth century. Tired of hearing it? Sorry, but discounting the medical facts isn't logical—it's called denial. We're all aware that smoking is dangerous, but let's take another look to reinforce our motivation.

Have you read any of the Surgeon General's warnings lately? "Smoking causes lung cancer, heart disease, emphysema, and may complicate pregnancy."

THE CHOICE IS YOURS

WHY I WANT OR NEED TO **QUIT SMOKING** | WHY I CHOOSE TO **CONTINUE SMOKING**

Reason:	Reason:
Result:	Result:
Reason:	Reason:
Result:	Result:
Reason:	Reason:
Result:	Result:
Reason:	Reason:
Result:	Result:
Reason:	Reason:
Result:	Result:
Reason:	Reason:
Result:	Result:
Reason:	Reason:
Result:	Result:
Reason:	Reason:
Result:	Result:
Reason:	Reason:
Result:	Result:
Reason:	Reason:
Result:	Result:
Reason:	Reason:
Result:	Result:

That tells only part of the story. The fact is, every year more Americans die from smoking-related diseases than from AIDS, alcohol, drug abuse, car accidents, firearms, toxic chemicals, or murder combined. At least one in every three smokers can expect to die prematurely from smoking, losing an average of 21 years of productive life. One out of every two adult smokers will develop a serious tobacco-related disease.

U.S. SMOKING-RELATED DEATHS IN 1996

Cancer	163,000
Coronary Heart Disease	135,000
Lung Disease	85,000
Stroke (brain attack)	23,000
Other (fires, vascular disease, accidents, etc.)	75,000
Total:	434,000

McGinnis, J. M., M.D., M.P.P., and Foege, W. H., M.D., M.D.H. "Actual Causes of Death in the United States." *Journal of American Medicine,* 1993; 270:2207–2212.

What Happens When You Smoke

Smoking is the underlying cause of one out of every three deaths that will occur in America today. One of the most potent human carcinogens any of us will ever encounter, tobacco smoke is responsible for stimulating 11 different kinds of cancer. Watching a previously healthy person cope with the debilitating effects of cancer or a paralyzed arm or leg resulting from a stroke is painful evidence of the high price we pay for the "freedom" to slowly kill ourselves by smoking. No one can smoke without some negative health consequence. After 10 or 15 years of smoking, destruction of lung tissues is clearly detectable. Since most Americans start smoking in their mid- to late teens, many young adults are already suffering from lung injury (emphysema and chronic bronchitis). Living with any of the chronic diseases caused by smoking is an agonizing existence.

Although most of us are familiar with these major consequences of smoking, here are some of the less frequently discussed health risks that may not have caught your attention:

- Impotence
- Osteoporosis (fragile bones that break easily)
- Spinal disc degeneration
- Blindness and cataracts, particularly in diabetics
- Facial wrinkling and premature aging of the skin
- Infertility
- Peptic ulcer disease
- Lower IQ in children of mothers who smoke
- More miscarriages, stillbirths, tubal pregnancies, low birthweight babies and sudden infant deaths in pregnant women who smoke
- Women who smoke during pregnancy increase their daughters' risk of miscarrying by 30 percent
- Men who smoke before conception increase their children's risk of childhood cancer
- Up to 40 percent of upper respiratory disorders in children are caused by breathing passive smoke from their adult caregivers
- Allergy and asthma attacks from secondhand smoke
- More complications following routine anesthesia and surgery
- Injury, including death, from cigarette-induced residential fires

How Nicotine Affects the Brain

The brain has several chemical "messengers" that carry signals from one part to another, telling it, in effect, how to feel. When nicotine enters the brain, it changes the levels of several of those messengers, thereby altering normal processes. When the chemical norepinephrine is stimulated by the arrival of nicotine, it sends a message of alertness, concentration, and heightened awareness. When nicotine disappears from the circulation, the brain experiences the opposite sensations, i.e., drowsiness and difficulty in concentrating.

Dopamine is another chemical messenger that is enhanced by nicotine. The signals that dopamine send go to the reward, or pleasure, center of the brain. Within 15 seconds of inhaling cigarette smoke, dopamine sends a message that makes the brain feel as if it's just sunk a basket from the back of the court.

Milligram for milligram, nicotine is the most potent addictive chemical to affect the human brain. When a smoker quits, the brain has to readjust to its normal chemistry, resulting in a post-nicotine slump that may be experienced as grumpiness, anger, or depression. These withdrawal symptoms can take anywhere from two to six weeks to wear off before the brain gets used to its normal chemistry again.

Many nonsmokers are unaware of these profound physiological effects— they just think smoking is a nasty, smelly habit that endangers both the smoker and nearby nonsmokers. But smoking is not just a psychological addiction, it's a physical one as well. For this reason, a serious and informed approach to quitting is crucial.

What Smoking "Type" Are You?

Before you quit smoking, it is very helpful to analyze your own unique bond with cigarettes. There are many reasons why people smoke, and understanding your own will give you valuable tools for success.

- Are you handcuffed to the habit of tobacco use as an unconscious routine, or out of boredom?
- Do you believe that the only effective way to deal with stress is to smoke?
- Have you started to think of yourself as a future ex-smoker yet?
- Finally, do you know how to help your body handle life without nicotine?

The Triangle of Nicotine Addiction

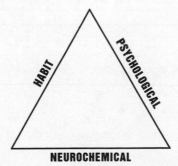

You must determine which of the three aspects of nicotine addiction— habit, psychological, or neurochemical—has the strongest hold on you. That way, you'll be able to replace what you get from smoking and stop the loss from becoming overwhelming. Taking the quiz on the following pages will help you see where you must work the hardest. Lack of preparation and failing to understand the real reasons behind your addiction are why 35 to 40 percent of people never make it past week one in the quitting process. Complete this quiz and combine the information with the results of the "Choices" exercise on page 18. You'll be armed with some compelling tools for a successful attack on your smoking habit.

Least Applies to Me/Most Applies to Me

A. I smoke cigarettes in order to keep myself from slowing down.

Never	Seldom	Average	Often	Always
①	②	③	④	⑤

B. Handling a cigarette is part of the enjoyment of smoking it.

Never	Seldom	Average	Often	Always
①	②	③	④	⑤

C. Smoking cigarettes is pleasant and relaxing.

Never	Seldom	Average	Often	Always
①	②	③	④	⑤

D. I light up a cigarette when I feel angry about something.

Never	Seldom	Average	Often	Always
①	②	③	④	⑤

E. When I run out of cigarettes, I find it almost unbearable until I can get more.

Never	Seldom	Average	Often	Always
①	②	③	④	⑤

F. I smoke cigarettes automatically without even being aware of it.

Never	Seldom	Average	Often	Always
①	②	③	④	⑤

G. I smoke cigarettes to stimulate myself, perk myself up.

Never	Seldom	Average	Often	Always
①	②	③	④	⑤

H. Part of the enjoyment of smoking a cigarette comes from the steps I take to light up.

Never	Seldom	Average	Often	Always
①	②	③	④	⑤

I. I find cigarettes pleasurable.

Never	Seldom	Average	Often	Always
1	2	3	4	5

J. When I feel uncomfortable or upset about something, I light up a cigarette.

Never	Seldom	Average	Often	Always
1	2	3	4	5

K. When I am not smoking a cigarette, I am very much aware of that fact.

Never	Seldom	Average	Often	Always
1	2	3	4	5

L. I light up a cigarette without realizing I still have one burning in the ashtray.

Never	Seldom	Average	Often	Always
1	2	3	4	5

M. I smoke cigarettes to give myself a lift.

Never	Seldom	Average	Often	Always
1	2	3	4	5

N. When I smoke a cigarette, part of the enjoyment is watching the smoke as I exhale it.

Never	Seldom	Average	Often	Always
1	2	3	4	5

O. I want a cigarette most when I am comfortable and relaxed.

Never	Seldom	Average	Often	Always
1	2	3	4	5

P. When I feel blue or want to take my mind off cares and worries, I smoke cigarettes.

Never	Seldom	Average	Often	Always
1	2	3	4	5

Q. I get a real gnawing hunger for a cigarette when I haven't smoked for a while.

Never	Seldom	Average	Often	Always
1	2	3	4	5

R. I've found a cigarette in my mouth and didn't remember putting it there.

Never	Seldom	Average	Often	Always
1	2	3	4	5

Scoring Your Test

Enter the number you circled over the appropriate space below. Line "A" is for question A, etc. Total the scores to the right.

A	+	G	+	M	=	_____
						Stimulation

B	+	H	+	N	=	_____
						Handling

C	+	I	+	O	=	_____
						Relaxation-Reward

D	+	J	+	P	=	_____
						Stress Reducer

E	+	K	+	Q	=	_____
						Craving

F	+	L	+	R	=	_____
						Habit

Throw Out the Old, Bring On the New

The highest scores indicate your strongest reasons for using tobacco (maximum 15 points). Now that you've identified yourself as a certain "type" of smoker, you can start to select healthy alternatives that will meet the same needs that were previously fulfilled by cigarettes. You may fall into more than one category; in that case, read all of the "type" descriptions that apply to you. Following are some suggestions based on your type; you may be able to come up with your own ideas as well.

Stimulation

IF THE FOLLOWING ARE TRUE:

- Cigarettes give you an increased sense of energy
- You begin the day with a cigarette
- You need that "little something" to keep you from slowing down during the day

• You feel good when you smoke and bad when you don't

TRY THIS REPLACEMENT BEHAVIOR INSTEAD:

• Find another source of stimulation, i.e., a safe substitute. Try a brisk walk, a little exercise, chewing sugarless gum, a new and fun hobby, playing with a pet, surfing the Internet, calling a friend.

Handling

IF THE FOLLOWING ARE TRUE:

• You enjoy manipulating the cigarette with your hands
• You make a production of lighting and holding a cigarette
• You enjoy watching the smoke as you exhale

TRY THIS REPLACEMENT BEHAVIOR INSTEAD:

• Pick something satisfying to manipulate other than a cigarette. Try a pen or pencil, take up doodling, write a story or poem, play with silly putty, finger a coin, piece of jewelry, or plastic straw. Indulge your creativity and start a "hands-on" hobby.

Relaxation-Reward

IF THE FOLLOWING ARE TRUE:

• You enhance pleasurable feelings by having a cigarette
• You enjoy a cigarette after dinner or with a drink
• You smoke as a reward

TRY THIS REPLACEMENT BEHAVIOR INSTEAD:

• Take a hard, honest look at the harmful effects of your habit—this may provide enough motivation. Or try other pleasurable pursuits such as going to a movie, renting a video, or mild physical activity like bowling or gardening. Take a hot bath, get a massage. Visualize yourself as a nonsmoker, enjoying all of the benefits.

Stress Reducer

IF THE FOLLOWING ARE TRUE:

• You light a cigarette when you are tense or angry
• You use a cigarette as a crutch

- You automatically light a cigarette when handling a personal problem
- You believe that smoking helps you deal with problems more effectively

TRY THIS REPLACEMENT BEHAVIOR INSTEAD:

- Anticipate stressful situations, and try to manage your life to remove pressure. Find new and exciting ways to reduce tension and let off emotional energy. Engage in 20 to 30 minutes of aerobic exercise, do some deep-breathing exercises, or study relaxation techniques such as guided imagery to create the sensation of a peaceful environment. Take a five-minute time-out instead of exploding in anger.

Craving

IF THE FOLLOWING ARE TRUE:

- You look forward to your next cigarette before finishing the one you are smoking
- You are constantly aware of when you are NOT smoking
- The time between each cigarette is a gradual buildup of pressure until you can have the next one

TRY THIS REPLACEMENT BEHAVIOR INSTEAD:

- Work to control your physical craving, which is based on how much nicotine your brain needs in order to feel comfortable. When the level dips too low, the brain sends reminders in the form of craving sensations. To break the cycle, wait two or three minutes before lighting a cigarette, and notice that the urge to smoke goes away. Cravings are a sort of chemical "alarm clock" that remind you when it's time to get another dose of nicotine. You can control these alarms by gradually reducing the amount you smoke. Alternatively, consider using medication such as nicotine replacement or Bupropion that helps break the chemical craving cycles. (See page 30 for more on medications.)

Habit

IF THE FOLLOWING ARE TRUE:

- You sometimes smoke a cigarette without realizing, or even wanting one
- You smoke automatically, without any satisfaction
- You sometimes find that you have lit two cigarettes

TRY THIS REPLACEMENT BEHAVIOR INSTEAD:

- Be aware at all times that you are using tobacco. Don't smoke in your usual place. Wrap each cigarette in paper to give yourself a reminder, and place them out of easy reach. Then ask yourself, "Do I really want this cigarette, or can I go without it?"

WHAT HAPPENS WHEN YOU QUIT

It's true that the negative aspects of smoking merit consideration—but so do the positive effects of quitting. Is there a former smoker anywhere who regrets that he or she was able to quit successfully? It's hard to imagine there is. Most often ex-smokers say, "What was I waiting for? If only I'd known how great it is to be free of smoking, I would have done this sooner!" But that doesn't mean quitting is easy—if that were the case, there would be no need for books like this.

The real miracle of quitting smoking is the amazing ability of the human body to recover after years of being constantly poisoned with toxins and chemicals from inhaling burning tobacco smoke. Below are some of the benefits you can expect after you successfully quit smoking. Remember, some of these effects take years to enact, so don't expect to return to perfect health after six nicotine-free months. Nicotine is an insidious poison that takes time to erase from the body, no matter how resilient you may be.

At 20 minutes after quitting

Blood pressure decreases
Pulse rate drops
Body temperature of hands and feet increases

At 8 hours

Carbon monoxide level in blood drops to normal

Oxygen level in blood increases to normal

At 24 hours

Chance of dying suddenly from a heart attack decreases

At 48 hours

Nerve endings start regrowing

Ability to smell and taste is enhanced

In the first week

Breathing becomes easier

Food has more flavor

Everything smells better

Start saving money that was burned up by smoking

In the first year

Improved lung function continues for up to five years

Heart disease risk is cut in half

First few years

Risk of bladder/cervical cancer is 50 percent lower

After 5 years

Risk of stroke/brain attack is similar to nonsmoker

Mouth/esophageal cancer risk is reduced by 50 percent

After 10 years

Lung cancer risk is reduced by one-third to one-half

After 15 years

Risk of heart disease/stroke is similar to nonsmoker

Lung cancer risk is reduced by 80 to 90 percent

These are generalities based on the average population. If you have an inherited risk of heart disease, cancer, stroke, or lung disease, then your chances are increased, making it even more important to stop playing with fire and stop smoking now. Your health-care provider can help you analyze your level of risk based on family history and your personal health habits.

Withdrawal Symptoms

Do you need nicotine to feel OK? Your brain may have become so used to your regular supply that it functions better with nicotine than without it. A nicotine-dependent brain will experience withdrawal symptoms when the nicotine supply it is accustomed to stops, but every person reacts differently. After quitting, some people may notice little change in how they feel, but others may suffer severe effects. Most smokers will experience at least four of the following symptoms when they go "nicotine-free" for 24 hours or more:

- Depressed mood
- Difficulty in sleeping
- Irritability
- Frustration
- Anger
- Anxiety
- Difficulty in concentrating
- Restlessness
- Increased appetite[1]

VISUALIZE THE GOAL:
A NICOTINE-FREE BRAIN

The transition to a healthy, nicotine-free brain may take only two weeks or last as long as six weeks for a few ex-smokers. If you can't bear living with the withdrawal symptoms and go back to smoking, then you are giving in to the destructive belief that you can't live without smoking.

CALL IN THE TROOPS: IF YOU CAN'T DO IT ALONE, GET HELP

For those who feel defeated by nicotine withdrawal symptoms, there is a way to ease the transition to a nicotine-free brain. The Agency for Health Care Policy and Research has issued a recommendation based on extensive studies by smoking cessation experts. Smokers who can't seem to quit on their own are urged to seek professional help in selecting medications that will reduce nicotine withdrawal symptoms. Enlisting the help of an experienced health-care professional, whether you elect to take medication or not, will dramatically improve your chances of success.

THE MEDICATIONS AND HOW THEY WORK

As we learned in Chapter 1, one of the effects of nicotine on the brain is to suppress the appetite. After years of smoking, sometimes as many as 35 or 40, the sudden return of a normal appetite when you quit can be overwhelming. A slower transition off nicotine can allow the brain to adjust little by little. Nicotine replacement works on this principle, and can be supplied in several different forms.

Nicotine Replacement

When you smoke, a high dose of nicotine enters the brain via an inhaled form, infiltrating its circulation in 15 seconds. Nicotine-replacement treatment supplies the brain with the nicotine it is used to from a non-tobacco source. Thus the user gets pure nicotine at a comfortable level without nicotine withdrawal symptoms. This marks the first, crucial transition point: no tobacco, only nicotine from now on. The nicotine levels are then gradually decreased and the user goes through a readjustment phase as the brain gets accustomed to lower doses. Finally, when treatment stops, the brain adjusts to the complete lack of nicotine and takes over the task of controlling its own chemical messengers. At this transition point, most new ex-smokers experience some degree of withdrawal symptoms, but others have no negative effects. This is the beginning of the nicotine-free experience. Unfortunately, after discontinuing nicotine replacement, some people suffer such troublesome symptoms that they relapse, returning to the nicotine source of choice, i.e., tobacco.

Four different forms of nicotine replacement are currently available. Each one delivers sufficient nicotine to the brain to satisfy the brain's craving for nicotine, but the amount is different for every person, and so treatment will vary. The most popular form is the skin patch, which delivers nicotine slowly and constantly right through the layers of the skin. Three brands are available over the counter, and a fourth is offered by prescription only. The next type of replacement therapy involves a gumlike substance, Nicorette, which is sold over the counter. The gum can be chewed slowly until a tingling sensation results. Nicotine enters the circulation through the lining of the mouth, and the gum is parked in the cheek until the next wave of nicotine craving arrives, when it can be chewed again.

The remaining two products both require a doctor's prescription. The newest one, the Nicotrol Inhaler, uses a menthol and nicotine vapor mixture in a device that looks like a straw or a filter on a cigar. The user "puffs" through the plastic mouthpiece whenever the craving strikes to receive a non-tobacco source of nicotine through the mouth lining, just as with the gum. The key benefit of absorbing nicotine through the lining of the mouth is that it does not enter the lungs. The user gets an adequate dose of nicotine without carbon monoxide or any of the other 4,800 chemicals (400 of them carcinogenic!) that are absorbed with every puff of tobacco.

The final option, nasal spray, delivers the highest dose of nicotine per use. One spray in each nostril supplies roughly the same amount of nicotine as one cigarette. Ask your doctor which of these nicotine replacement devices is right for you, and be sure to read the package inserts to make sure there are no contraindications that may apply to you.

Bupropion Hydrochloride (Zyban)

In 1997, an oral tablet named Bupropion (Zyban) became the first non-nicotine medication to be approved in the United States as an aid in smoking cessation. Bupropion affects the brain's pleasure and rewards center, just like nicotine (in the late 1980s Bupropion was used as a prescription anti-depressant); but unlike nicotine, it does not stimulate a high release of dopamine and norepinephrine. Thus it is not addictive. Bupropion acts to keep a constant balance between these brain chemicals, preventing the sudden low levels of chemicals that can cause craving and withdrawal symptoms.

There are three phases to taking a course of Bupropion. In the first phase, the smoker takes a pill once or twice a day for one or two weeks prior to officially quitting. He or she then sets a quit date, at which point the medication should be working in optimum mode. During this period, smokers often state that smoking seems "less satisfying" or "doesn't taste as good" as before; in addition, the length of time between cravings may increase and their intensity lessen. Many smokers voluntarily reduce the number of cigarettes they smoke during this preparation phase because of Bupropion's effect on the brain chemistry.

In the second phase after stopping tobacco, Bupropion eases the effects of nicotine withdrawal symptoms by preventing the rapid changes in chemical levels in the brain that would normally occur. After a few weeks when nicotine withdrawal is over, the third phase takes over, the brain adjusts back to its regular functioning with its normal, fluctuating levels of natural mood-changing chemicals. At that point, the smoker will no longer feel the need for Bupropion. When the medication is stopped, there are no withdrawal symptoms because the brain has regained its balance and is back on "autopilot."

Bupropion must be prescribed by a physician, and he or she will want to know about any past history of depression or anxiety you may have, particularly if it required medical treatment. Unless there are contraindications, your doctor can advise you on how to use Bupropion.

A recent multicenter study[2] examined the quit rates of smokers in three groups. One used only Bupropion, another used only the nicotine patch, and a third group used a combination of both Bupropion and the patch. While each treatment was effective compared to placebo, those on Bupropion had significantly higher quit rates than the group on the patch. Subjects who used both Bupropion and the patch in combination showed only slightly higher quit rates at nine weeks and after one year than those who used Bupropion alone. The findings from this study imply that combining the two medications may not be necessary for all smokers.

Due to the increased costs, the combination of both the Bupropion and the patch is not routinely recommended for everyone until one medication alone has failed to give successful results. Your doctor can help you determine whether you may do better with the nicotine patch, with Bupropion, or with both.

Less Weight Gain with Medication

Four out of six smoking cessation studies show that using nicotine gum produces less weight gain than a "cold turkey" effort without medication.[3] When the ex-smoker gives up nicotine gum, however, the brain is again left without the control that nicotine exerts on the appetite, and some weight gain may occur unless he or she changes old eating and exercise habits. Similar studies on Bupropion also show a decreased tendency for users to gain weight.[4] This is not surprising, since Bupropion has long been known as an antidepressant that suppresses appetite, as nicotine does. But as with nicotine gum, once Bupropion is stopped, weight gain will need to be controlled in other ways. Of course, once you've conquered the addiction to nicotine it becomes easier to focus on improving your eating and exercise habits to maintain a healthy weight.

Smokers who are concerned about excessive weight gain may want to consult a health-care professional and request a program on either nicotine replacement or Bupropion. These medications should be used alongside the Personal Nutrition Management Plan in Chapter 5 to prevent weight gain after the medications are stopped. Why not use every advantage available in the struggle to return to a healthy, controllable appetite and a smoke-free existence?

THIS IS THE BOTTOM LINE on using these proven medications in a stop-smoking program. They:
- are effective
- improve quitting rates
- are cheaper than the cost of smoking
- reduce nicotine withdrawal symptoms when used properly
- appear to reduce weight gain associated with the early months of smoking cessation
- are safer than the risks of continued smoking

WATCH OUT FOR BOOBY TRAPS: WHEN YOU NEED PROFESSIONAL HELP

We have already seen how the nicotine-dependent brain can swing out of control when nicotine is withdrawn and levels of mood-changing chemicals drop drastically. By taking the quiz on page 22 you have learned how to replace some of your needs from nicotine with healthier alternatives. There are some psychological conditions, however, that can sabotage even the best-laid plans to quit. Many of the failures by people resolutely determined and highly motivated to stop smoking can be explained by the existence of one of these disorders.

Psychological Conditions Affected by Nicotine

- anxiety
- panic disorders
- manic-depressive (bipolar) disorder
- depression
- family history of suicide attempt
- post-traumatic stress disorder
- chemical dependency (alcohol, illicit drugs)
- schizophrenia
- eating disorders (anorexia or bulimia)
- attention deficit disorder

The good news is that all of these conditions are treatable. If you or a family member are afflicted, discuss the situation with your doctor prior to your quit date so you can get help before attempting to stop smoking. A failed quit attempt will cause lack of self-confidence, so it's wise to get yourself into optimum physical and mental condition first. Your doctor will be able to advise you on managing first the medical problem and then later, the problem of nicotine dependence.

In a study of smoking and depression, only one in six nonsmokers questioned revealed the presence of depression, whereas one in three smokers showed depressive symptoms.[5] For people who think they can't live without nicotine, getting effective treatment for anxiety or depression may help them quit smoking with much less difficulty.[6]

The following case history illuminates this interaction: Jim, in his forties, was a successful, happily married district attorney, very involved in sports and fitness. He had tried three times, unsuccessfully, to quit smoking: once in college, once after finishing law school, and recently using the nicotine patch. Within weeks of quitting, Jim always experienced a dark cloud descending over his emotions, and was placed on antidepressants twice. Even on the low-dose patch, with a dose of nicotine that was evidently too low for him, his brain chemistry dipped into depression. When Jim eventually started smoking again, it was clear to him that his mood improved greatly within a matter of days. Jim honestly wanted to quit, yet felt physically trapped. His family had a history of depression and chemical dependency; in his case, nicotine was his "over the counter antidepressant." But he sensed it was slowly killing him, even though smoking daily kept him feeling fine.

Jim's treatment provided him with the stability he needed in order to recover from nicotine dependence. He was pretreated for two weeks with Bupropion, which, as we have seen, works in a similar way to nicotine. After setting a quit date, he added a nicotine patch and successfully stayed off cigarettes for about four weeks. Since his mood was greatly improved on the Bupropion compared to his third quit attempt, when he had tried the patch alone, he continued with the Bupropion alone for another two months. Jim has now been nicotine-free for five years and has experienced no further episodes of depression.

In Jim's case, simply stabilizing his brain chemistry with Bupropion during the initial weaning off the nicotine patch did the job. Other people may have a stronger tendency toward depression, and may need to take an antidepressant for a longer period under a doctor's care.

DON'T START QUITTING
UNTIL YOU'RE READY

When you set out to succeed at something important, you anticipate some hard work and possibly an occasional setback, but you don't give up until you've reached your goal. Unfortunately with most smokers, a decision to quit often ends in failure. The best tactic is to devise a specific program tailored to your own needs and then stray from it as little as possible. If you know what to expect and prepare your responses ahead of time, you can avoid many of the negative consequences. The process will be easier if you enlist the help of a professional counselor or health-care provider.

Get All The Pieces on The Table

This book provides you with the tools to understand the reasons why you smoke and to identify your personal barriers to quitting. If you have never made a serious effort to quit smoking and want this to be your last attempt, then put the pieces together as follows:

• **ARM YOURSELF WITH INFORMATION:** In addition to this book, you may find it helpful to consult other well-balanced "How to stop smoking" books. (See appendix page 297.) Use all the information in these books to make a customized plan that will suit your needs.

• **GET THE SUPPORT YOU NEED:** Find a buddy who will "be there" for you—in person or by telephone—when you find yourself wavering. The best buddies are those who have themselves successfully quit smoking since they understand what you are facing and can offer incentive, but any supportive, level-headed friend will do. Contact volunteer agencies such as the American Lung Association, Nicotine Anonymous, or your local hospital to find out when the next support meeting will take place. If your state has a free telephone helpline, you can talk with a trained counselor when you need encouragement. Check the source guide on page 289 for Web sites and chat rooms dealing with the subject. (These are helpful for late night cravings when no one else is up in your time zone!)

• **CONSULT A HEALTH-CARE PROFESSIONAL:** For an even better chance at quitting permanently, talk with a doctor about the possibility of using medications before you quit. Mention concerns that you have about past failures due to factors such as mood swings or weight gain. If you opt for medication, fit it around the timing of your quit date to give yourself the best chance at success. Keep your doctor apprised of any problems as they occur, before they have a chance to get out of hand.

Getting help may seem complicated, but why play around when the consequences of failure leave so much at stake? The benefits of living smoke-free are so inviting, and so realistically attainable. So gather all the resources you may conceivably need and join the 50 million Americans who have already decided to "make smoking history."

QUITTING ENVY: WHEN YOUR FRIENDS AREN'T HELPING

If you have family members or friends who smoke, consider the possibility that they may become threatened by your positive progress toward quitting. Your decision will put pressure on them to follow, and they may not yet be ready to take the plunge. Be diplomatic, and keep the focus on your own recovery rather than comparing yourself with others. Don't let their comments derail you from your journey. Be prepared for some changes in your relationships with smoking friends when you no longer share the "dark and reckless, dangerous pleasures" of being smoking buddies. You may be prepared for your own inner struggle with the demon nicotine, but not for friendly fire. Be sure their "envy" doesn't catch you unaware.

GET YOURSELF A WHOLE NEW ATTITUDE

When you were a smoker, you may have been an advocate of "smokers' rights," namely, the right to light up anywhere without interference. Remember that as a smoker, you had no choice but to smoke, and that sounds a little like slavery.

Instead, try out a new version of smokers' rights: "I have the right to choose whether I smoke or not." Now THAT'S freedom.

CHAPTER 3
Coping with Cravings After Smoking Cessation

After a day or two without cigarettes, you'll probably notice a few changes already taking place in your body. You might be aware of the gradual heightening of your senses of smell and taste, along with increased circulation in your fingertips and toes. While these effects vary depending on how much you smoked, how long you smoked, and how physically active you are, one change most new ex-smokers consistently notice is a strong urge to eat. Food cravings are partly the desire to replace the habit of smoking with another activity, but primarily they stem from a physical need to satisfy a hunger that smoking and nicotine diminished.

If you give into the cravings and binge on sugar, starch, and fat, the nasty symptoms of nicotine withdrawal will be temporarily eased. Unfortunately, if you choose the wrong foods—that is, foods high in calories from fat and sugar—you're likely to start on a downward spiral in which you overeat, feel fine for a while, then feel worse and return for another snack. Even though it's reassuring to know that certain foods can make your cravings go away, in your new nonsmoking world you need to be careful not to substitute one addiction—cigarettes—for another—food. This chapter will help you understand the physical basis of your cravings so you can work with those feelings and find healthy ways to satisfy hunger and avoid weight gain. At the end of this chapter you'll find a list of new, improved eating rules—designed specifically for the new ex-smoker—that will help you reach those goals.

A BIOLOGICAL BASIS FOR CRAVINGS

Nicotine affects the release of certain chemicals in the brain—norepinephrine, dopamine, and serotonin—that trigger appetite. One puff from a cigarette usually momentarily satisfies the nicotine addiction, but since the sensation of hunger feels very similar to the desire for a cigarette, smoking also effectively squelches the smoker's desire for food.

All this changes the moment you quit smoking. Without the steady stream of nicotine, chemical reactions in your body and brain begin to function normally again and your appetite returns to normal. Part of your craving is just the return of your normal appetite, which was effectively suppressed with each cigarette you smoked. But it's important to remember that appetite is a GOOD thing—it encourages us to eat, which keeps our bodies running. Unfortunately, however, our appetites don't always discriminate. We gravitate toward tasty foods that are high in fat and sugar. It's up to us to remain vigilant and select a healthy diet of carbohydrates, proteins, "good" fats, vitamins, minerals, and fiber.

FOOD AND MOOD

Scientists have recently discovered that neurotransmitters in the brain can have a profound effect on our mood, energy level, and eating and sleep patterns. They've also identified certain chemicals that switch the brain's hunger sensors on and off like a light switch. Four neurotransmitters that are sensitive to food intake and changes in dietary patterns are serotonin, NPY (neuropeptide Y), galanin, and endorphins. If we understand how each of these chemicals affects our appetite and the satisfaction of our hunger, we can work with that knowledge to control our cravings.

THE ROLE OF SEROTONIN

Serotonin is a mood enhancer and stabilizer. A protein produced in the brain, it has a strong positive effect on our sense of calmness, peace, and emotional stability. Low serotonin levels may result in insomnia, depression, and food cravings. Serotonin can be a powerful ally to the new ex-smoker. By eating foods that keep serotonin levels relatively high, you can satisfy your appetite— and ease your cravings—without resorting to sudden, destructive binges.

Serotonin is manufactured from an amino acid called tryptophan, found in protein-rich foods such as turkey, meats, dairy products, and fish, in conjunction with vitamins B_6, B_{12}, and other nutrients. Scientists have discovered that a diet high in carbohydrates, i.e., whole-grain breads, cereals, rice, fruits, and vegetables, can also boost our serotonin levels.

Ironically, eating a protein-rich meal *lowers* the tryptophan and serotonin levels in the brain, while eating a carbohydrate-rich snack does just the opposite. Tryptophan shares an entry gate into the brain with several other large amino acids, such as tyrosine. When you eat a high-protein meal, you flood the blood with amino acids that block the entry of tryptophan and serotonin into the brain. As a result, your serotonin levels might actually fall, causing you to feel irritable, have trouble sleeping, or start craving food.

According to *Food & Mood* by Elizabeth Somer, M.A., R.D. (Henry Holt, 1999), if you feed your cravings with high-carbohydrate foods, such as a dessert or starch, you might momentarily boost your serotonin levels and satisfy your need—but the feeling won't last. A carbohydrate-rich meal triggers the release of insulin from the pancreas, causing most amino acids floating in the blood to be absorbed into the body's cells—except tryptophan, which remains in the bloodstream at relatively high levels. With the competition removed, tryptophan freely enters the brain, causing serotonin levels to rise. The high serotonin levels in turn increase your feelings of calmness or drowsiness, improve your sleep patterns, and reduce your cravings.

But this carbohydrate binge sets off a seesaw effect on your appetite. For your next meal, you'll probably select high-protein, lower-carbohydrate foods, such as a turkey or tuna sandwich, perhaps with a glass of milk. These foods effectively reduce your serotonin levels, likely causing you to become jittery or depressed, which combined with your nicotine-withdrawal anxiety, leaves you once again at the mercy of your cravings. And so you swing back and forth from carbohydrates to proteins throughout the day, in part because of fluctuations in your neurotransmitters. Studies show that people who crave carbohydrates often as well as obese people have chronically lower serotonin levels than people who prefer protein-rich snacks or thin people. Their extra-low serotonin levels leave them feeling anxious, irritable—and constantly craving a serotonin "fix."

The following specifies how different food components affect serotonin:

- **SUGAR:** Triggers a quick release of insulin, which lowers blood levels of most large amino acids and increases blood levels of tryptophan. Results in a short-term increase in brain serotonin levels.

- **STARCH:** Triggers a slow release of insulin, which lowers blood levels of most large amino acids and increases blood levels of tryptophan. The result is a long-term increase in brain serotonin levels. Processed grains can have a more dramatic effect on insulin and blood sugar levels, resulting in short-term increases in serotonin levels. (For a complete discussion of unprocessed and processed grains, see page 57.)

- **VITAMIN B$_6$:** Aids in the manufacture of serotonin. A deficiency of vitamin B$_6$ reduces serotonin production, affecting mood and food cravings.

- **ESTROGEN:** Inhibits vitamin B$_6$ status and decreases brain serotonin levels through its effect on NPY.

- **TRYPTOPHAN:** Increases brain serotonin levels when combined with vitamins B$_6$ and B$_{12}$, folic acid, and other nutrients.

- **PROTEIN:** Raises blood levels of large amino acids and decreases blood levels of tryptophan. Results in a decrease in brain serotonin levels and an increase in carbohydrate cravings.

- **FAT:** There is no documented effect of fat on serotonin levels.[1]

MORE INSULIN IN THE BLOOD

In addition to the serotonin seesaw, new ex-smokers have a second battle to face: a craving for sweets, which is amplified by increased levels of insulin in their bodies. Insulin, with the help of chromium, magnesium, and other nutrients, allows blood sugar to pass from the bloodstream into the cells of the body, supplying energy to the tissues and maintaining normal blood sugar levels. In 1988, Dr. Neil Grunberg's lab at the Uniformed Services University in Bethesda, Maryland, discovered that nicotine lowers blood insulin levels. Therefore when a smoker suddenly quits, higher levels of insulin begin to circulate throughout his or her bloodstream, resulting in an increased craving for sweets—in addition to the return of the normal appetite. According to Judith Rodin, Ph.D., professor of psychology and psychiatry at the University of Pennsylvania, people are hungriest and want sweets the most when their insulin levels are high.

HOW BLOOD SUGAR CONTROLS APPETITE AND MOOD

Blood sugar is probably the most important factor relating to appetite and mood control. Many hormones, including glucagon from the pancreas, epinephrine and the glucocorticoids from the adrenal glands, and thyroxine from the thyroid gland, are involved in raising blood sugar levels when they fall below normal concentrations. In contrast, insulin balances the effects by lowering blood sugar levels when they get too high.

Here's how insulin works. During digestion, sugars and starches are broken down into their simple units of glucose or fructose. These simple sugars enter the bloodstream and trigger the release of insulin from the pancreas. Insulin, along with other nutrients, allows blood sugar to enter the cells and supply energy to the tissues. When nicotine enters the system, it lowers insulin levels, causing you to feel less hungry. The equation is simple: Eliminate nicotine and your insulin level rises, thus stimulating your appetite. At the end of this chapter you'll find simple dietary tips to help you counteract the cravings for sweets produced by high levels of insulin.

THE APPETITE CONTROL CENTER

While the foods you eat can affect your mood, so too can several chemical messengers produced by the hypothalamus, which is the appetite control center of your brain. Long-term excessive dieting—or even overnight fasting—triggers the release of two appetite-stimulating neurotransmitters, NPY and galanin, so if you confront your new cravings by starving yourself, your body will respond by producing even more NPY and galanin. Since these neuro-

transmitters effectively stimulate hunger, your cravings won't go away—
they'll only get worse.

Higher insulin levels, lower serotonin levels, increased production of
NPY and galanin: The new ex-smoker is faced with a great deal of chemical
pressure to *eat food now,* making it nearly impossible to avoid the temptation
to binge. That's why it's so important to listen to your appetite and adjust
your diet during these crucial early days. The goal is to counteract the biological basis for cravings, and the food plan in Chapter 5 can help you avoid
extreme dieting—and extreme bingeing.

HOW NPY AFFECTS APPETITE

NPY, along with blood glucose levels, serotonin, and other chemicals, boosts
your desire for carbohydrate-rich foods. According to Sarah Leibowitz, Ph.D.,
a professor of neurobiology at Rockefeller University in New York City, as
NPY levels go up, so does your craving for sweet or starchy foods. When Dr.
Leibowitz injected NPY into the hypothalamus of animals, she observed that
they immediately chose carbohydrates over fatty foods. She also found a direct
link between her animals' desire for carbohydrates and their NPY levels: The
higher the NPY level, the more they wanted carbohydrates. Conversely, as
soon as they indulged in carbohydrates, their NPY levels began to decrease.

NPY works by jump-starting our eating cycle in the morning. Sugar
stores (glycogen) in the muscles and liver are drained overnight, and when we
wake, waning blood sugar levels send a message to the brain to release NPY.
This may be why we gravitate toward carbohydrate-rich foods, such as cereal,
toast, or bagels, when we wake up. (This may also explain why food cravings
intensify during and after dieting or food restriction; stress and strict dieting
trigger the appetite center to produce more NPY.) Probably a survival mechanism, NPY forces us to get more quick-energy carbohydrates into the system.

As a new ex-smoker, if you ignore the feelings that your increased NPY
stimulates in the morning, you run the risk of bingeing on a bag of cookies
in the afternoon. It's much more sensible to listen to your appetite and eat
properly. Dietitians have long alerted their patients to a simple truth: Deny-
ing hunger pangs leads to weight gain, and NPY is the chemical behind this
pattern.

FAT CRAVINGS

Different neurotransmitters affect our desire for carbohydrates, sugar, and protein in different ways, but what about our urges for fat? A specific set of chemical messengers from the hypothalamus, including galanin and the endorphins, affects our fat cravings. Research shows that as our galanin levels rise, so does our desire for foods that contain fat—so the more galanin we produce, the more fat we eat. Likewise, when galanin is injected into the hypothalamus of laboratory animals, they select fat-laden foods over carbohydrate-rich choices.

Scientists have also known about various drugs that "turn off" galanin activity and reduce our cravings for fat. Nicotine appears to be one of those drugs. According to Dr. Neil Grunberg, professor of psychology and neuroscience at the Uniformed Services University of the Health Sciences, nicotine decreases galanin levels in some strains of female rats. When nicotine is taken away, the animals' galanin levels rise—and so does their desire for fatty foods.

According to Dr. Leibowitz, whereas NPY levels are highest in the morning, galanin kicks in about midafternoon. This could explain why we go from wanting bagels and pancakes in the morning—as quick-energy fuel after a night of fasting—to wanting a hamburger with the works in the afternoon or evening. Our preference for fatty foods later in the day is possibly the body's attempt to store up long-term energy in anticipation of the overnight fast.

THE GALANIN ROLLER COASTER

The unique—and risky—thing about galanin is that the more fat you eat, the more galanin your body makes, and the more fat you crave. If you overindulge with a high-fat meal at lunch, you'll end up craving more fat the rest of the day. It's very important for new ex-smokers to understand the biological causes for these cravings as they must learn to satisfy this hormone very carefully. The key is to eat some fat, but not too much.

ENDORPHINS

Fat and nicotine both release another type of chemical into the brain called endorphins. Endorphins energize the mind and lift the spirits—like the feeling of euphoria that long-distance runners experience after a good workout.

Endorphins directly stimulate the appetite. When laboratory animals are injected with a medication that increases endorphin levels, they eat more. Endorphins may also work in combination with galanin to trigger strong cravings for sweet and creamy foods. When you quit smoking, you immediately cut off one of your body's prime sources of endorphins. It's only natural that you'll look to satisfy this biological need for endorphins in other ways—and the most obvious, and tastiest, source is fatty foods.

GIRLS (AND BOYS) JUST WANNA HAVE FUN

This strong desire to substitute one source of pleasure for another is played out again with sugar. Independent of serotonin, nicotine is known to stimulate the pleasure center in the brain in much the same way sugar does. Active smokers crave sweets much less than ex-smokers, but when nicotine is removed from their systems, they immediately seek a substitute and settle on sugar. Sugar stimulates norepinephrine in the sympathetic nervous system and promotes a sense of arousal; much like nicotine, it increases the heart rate, boosts energy levels, and rushes more oxygen to the brain. The bottom line is that sugar makes you feel good. Also, as new ex-smokers will freely admit, sugar is a common way to counteract the nicotine withdrawal symptoms that make them feel bad.

WHAT ABOUT CHOCOLATE?

Indeed, the most powerful food cravings new ex-smokers experience are for sugar and fat *combinations*—and the most powerful sugar and fat combination is chocolate. Chocolate has the ability to stimulate the dopamine pleasure centers in the brain in much the same way caffeine and nicotine do. But chocolate is not as potent; it takes a lot of chocolate to duplicate the lift you get from smoking a single cigarette. Some new ex-smokers try to substitute large quantities of chocolate for cigarettes to boost the sagging dopamine levels left behind when they stopped receiving their daily dose of nicotine. Be sure to avoid this trap. Chocolate addictions are real.

NEW, IMPROVED EATING RULES

If you can eat just a small portion of sugar or fat to calm down, and you're committed to working *with* your cravings—as opposed to dieting and binge-ing—you're ready to follow a few new, improved eating rules. These simple food guidelines, created specifically for the new ex-smoker, work to stabilize the mood and smooth out the peaks and valleys caused by nicotine withdrawal. Their goal is to help you satisfy your cravings without gaining weight.

• Eat Every 2 to 4 Hours

If you go four or five hours without eating, free fatty acids are released into the bloodstream, breaking down fat and creating a fasting situation. The hypothalamus then releases chemicals such as NPY to let your body know it's hungry. It's a survival mechanism, but one you can control.

If you make the mistake of waiting until you're starving before you eat, your body has already told your brain that it's hungry. This triggers the urge to overeat. Plan ahead, eat frequently, and make sure that you never become ravenous. This is especially relevant when the body is under stress, such as the first few weeks directly after smoking cessation.

• Eat Breakfast

In terms of stabilizing your brain chemistry, the worst thing you can do is skip meals altogether. If you miss breakfast in particular, NPY continues to escalate, so that by the afternoon you don't want just a small portion of carbohydrates, you want the entire bag of cookies. We always knew that breakfast skippers tended to eat more calories later in the day and weigh more than breakfast eaters; now there's a chemical explanation for that observation.

• Spread Out Your Calories

An effective way to respond to erratic blood sugars is to eat smaller, more frequent meals. If this works for you, remember that it's important to distribute your calories throughout the day rather than add more calories to each meal. In other words, spread out your portions, and don't simply increase them as you increase the number of times you eat.

If you're inclined to eat salad, spaghetti, and bread for dinner, try eating the bread, or substituting a cracker or cookie for the bread, in the midafternoon. The reverse is also true: If you like a starchy snack in the midafternoon as a serotonin booster, eat less starch at dinner. And if there's a specific time of day when you're very susceptible to cravings, try carrying healthy snacks with you. A banana or a Ziploc bag containing ¼ cup of nuts, for example, is an easy, healthy, and convenient way to satisfy your hunger without overloading on calories.

• Emphasize Unprocessed Foods

Virtually all carbohydrates are broken down or converted to glucose. Whether it's a candy bar, a bowl of oatmeal, or a plate of broccoli, the carbohydrates in these foods will end up in your bloodstream as glucose. Different types of glucose, however, cause different chemical changes in your body and affect your mood in different ways. When you're confronting the stress of smoking cessation, it's important to eat those foods containing carbohydrates that help you maintain a stable mood so you can avoid artificial highs and lows.

Candy bars contain simple sugars that cause a rapid rise in glucose levels, resulting in a temporary "sugar high." The simple sugars trigger insulin production, which begins pulling glucose out of the bloodstream and bringing glucose levels back to normal. But as excess insulin is secreted, glucose levels slip below normal, causing you to feel drained and lethargic. So, although simple sugars can give you a quick burst of energy, you'll probably end up feeling more tired and sluggish shortly after you eat them. In contrast, complex carbohydrates, especially whole grains, cause a slow, gradual rise in blood glucose levels. They allow you to avoid the extremes of "sugar highs" followed by "sugar lows." During the extra-stressful time of confronting nicotine withdrawal, eating those foods that can help stabilize your mood might make the difference between bingeing on a bag of cookies—or even breaking your commitment and reaching for a cigarette.

One very effective and healthy way to satisfy your cravings is to eat foods that have been minimally processed. In doing so, not only will you avoid wildly fluctuating blood sugar levels, but you will probably eat fewer calories as well. One reason: Unprocessed foods don't leave a lot of room in your stomach for junk. In addition, foods in their whole, natural state automatically take care of your fiber needs, boost serotonin levels, and keep blood sugar levels stable. Consider the spectrum of carbohydrates: Whole grains (oats, rice, wheat kernels) are the best to balance out blood sugar; refined grains (white bread, pasta) tend to stabilize blood sugar levels a little better; while sugar, as you know by now, is the worst. Eat a bowl of oatmeal instead of a granola bar, a baked potato instead of potato chips, or corn on the cob instead of high-fructose corn syrup.

• Remember the 5-a-Day Fruit and Vegetable Rule

Another simple way to satisfy cravings and keep blood sugar in check is to eat plenty of fruits and vegetables. Try eating two fruits and/or two vegetables at every meal and one portion of either every time you snack. The benefits to this are many: You'll get a good dose of vitamins, minerals, and fiber; you'll boost serotonin levels; and you'll keep your blood sugar levels stable.

• Get Vegetables from Soups

A pot of well-seasoned broth, stocked with vegetables, meats, or seafood, is a delicious way to get your vitamins, minerals, and fiber—all essential nutrients to the person going through nicotine withdrawal. A creamy puree of your favorite vegetable—broccoli, sweet potato, or carrot, for example—is another wonderful way to get your allotment.

• Respond to Your Cravings

The best way to manage food cravings is by satisfying them immediately—but with small portions. Abstinence and restriction only fuel cravings, trigger binges, and harm emotions. You'll end up feeling hungry and depressed, which is not the optimum frame of mind for someone confronting the rigors of nicotine withdrawal. The conclusion: Food cravings are not a problem to be treated, but a blessing to be encouraged. Of course, we all want to avoid those "don't even start" foods, which taste so good and satisfy our needs so fully that we have a hard time controlling our portions.

• Eat Complex Carbohydrates Along with Sweets

When we satisfy our cravings with sugary foods, we do feel better, but only until the moment our blood sugar drops. You can get the same serotonin benefit—without the roller coaster ride—by choosing whole grains or complex carbohydrates at each meal. If you still have a craving for sweets, a small amount will satisfy you. When your sweet tooth comes in the midafternoon, it could be a call for a serotonin boost to improve your mood. Try eating a piece of whole-grain toast with honey or jam, or have some lightly sugared whole-grain cereal. These food choices will help lift your serotonin levels gradually so you can avoid a blood sugar crash.

• Work in the Chocolate

If it's chocolate you crave, have it at the end of the meal rather than as a meal replacement. In her book *Food & Mood,* Elizabeth Somer suggests making a chocolate fondue. Cut up 2 cups of fresh fruit, then portion out ¼ cup of fat-free chocolate syrup, and dip each piece of fruit in the syrup. This will help you spread your chocolate fix out for 30 minutes, and you'll be eating mostly mood-elevating, health-enhancing fruit.

• Eat Fat—But Not Too Much

At lunchtime, make sure you satisfy the neurotransmitter galanin very gently. If you ignore it, you won't be satisfied; but if you overindulge, you'll stimulate your fat cravings for the rest of the day. Have a turkey sandwich with mustard or a tuna fish sandwich with a small amount of mayonnaise. Refer to the menus on page 79 for more great lunch ideas.

CONTROLLING CRAVINGS

The cravings you have when you quit smoking are strong biological forces. Research into neurotransmitters and other appetite-controlling processes is only 20 years old, but it's already had a profound effect on how new ex-smokers confront their symptoms of nicotine withdrawal. Given the research, the idea that you can use willpower alone to control cravings is illogical and outdated.

Now that you understand a little more about the biological basis for your cravings, and know how to integrate your cravings into healthy meals, you're ready to move on to a complete nutritional blueprint for a smoke-free lifestyle. The personal nutrition plans in the next two chapters contain guidelines designed to calm you down, help you stay off tobacco, and meet your nutritional needs—all without going overboard on calories.

CHAPTER 4
Ten Steps:
Eating for Health

Make sure you don't gain weight when you stop smoking by following the 10 steps outlined here *before* you quit. If you've already quit, still study these steps before going on to Chapter 5, since they contain important information that applies to you as well.

No matter how old or how physically fit you are, quitting smoking will improve your health. Without inhaling cigarette smoke into your lungs on a regular basis, you'll almost certainly be lowering your risk of contracting some types of cancer, lowering your blood pressure, and reducing your risk of heart and lung disease. If you couple smoking cessation with a change of diet and achieve your optimum weight, your health can continue to improve even further—and you'll feel great! This means making a serious commitment not only to quitting smoking, but also to eating properly and exercising regularly. It means learning to enjoy healthy foods in a society of abundance, and learning to make wise food choices despite the stress that life will bring, particularly during the difficult early period of nicotine withdrawal. And it means never forgetting that you're making the right choice.

AVOID FAD DIETS

If you're feeling anxious or even desperate about the possibility of gaining weight after you quit smoking, you might be tempted to try the latest fad diet. It's hard to pick up a newspaper or magazine these days without encountering an ad or story touting some amazing new weight-loss discovery:

new foods and supplements, special programs promoting fast weight loss, or even medications to reduce the appetite. These diets are appealing because they promise quick and effortless weight loss, but if you've tried them, you've probably discovered that they come with hidden costs. Weight loss using these approaches typically results in weight gain as soon as you return to your old eating habits. Ultimately, going on and off fad diets might even be harmful to your overall health because yo-yo dieting decreases your metabolism and trains your body to store fat cells more efficiently.

The best solution for the new ex-smoker is to make an immediate transition from the ritual, habit, and addiction of cigarette smoking to a new, healthy lifestyle that includes exercise, eating regularly, and making nutritious food choices. It's also important to develop a positive attitude that helps you think and behave in a way that supports all of your efforts. (We offer different solutions for long-term ex-smokers—people who've already successfully quit cigarettes—in the next chapter.)

What follows is a 10-step plan designed to help you achieve this new, beneficial lifestyle. It combines diet, exercise, and new ways of thinking about food and eating in a program that you can tailor to your particular needs. Although not a diet in the strict sense of the word, it does provide you with nutritional guidelines, menu plans for the home and on the go, and healthy recipes that incorporate your favorite foods. But unlike other nondiet approaches, you'll find here the structure you need to make sensible choices based on the foods you like and the life you lead. By incorporating these 10 simple steps into your new nonsmoking lifestyle, you'll have the best chance of avoiding weight gain, as well as the real possibility of losing weight after quitting.

It's been said that you are what you eat. Your diet not only affects what you weigh, but also your health and emotional well-being. Smokers tend to have lower levels of certain vitamins and minerals in their blood—which can create or aggravate specific health problems—as well as higher levels of cholesterol or triglycerides, which can increase the risk of heart attacks or strokes. The 10 steps that follow are designed to help new ex-smokers control their weight *and* regain their health.

If you're concerned about gaining weight right after you stop smoking, these steps will help prevent that. And here's more good news—your new diet may not require a major overhaul; with most people, only a handful of foods do the greatest damage. For these ex-smokers, the most radical dietary changes might consist of cutting back on rich desserts, replacing lunchtime burgers and fries with turkey sandwiches and soup, and eating smaller portions of bread and pasta with dinner. Once these changes are implemented, new ex-smokers are well on the way to controlling their calorie intake.

EATING FOR HEALTH

• **STEP 1:** Avoid getting overly hungry. Don't skip meals. Eat at least three or four times a day.

HERE'S WHY If you thought you were cutting calories by opting for coffee and cigarettes instead of breakfast, it's time for a change. Breakfast skippers tend to have more body fat and to eat more calories at other meals throughout the day. And never postpone lunch or dinner until you become ravenous—that's a definite trigger to overeat.

HERE'S HOW
- Follow the menu plans in this book.
- Shop at least once a week to make sure you always have the fixings for quick and easy meals on hand.
- Carry snacks of fruit and crackers. For a complete list of snacks, see page 127.

• **STEP 2:** Have chicken and fish for dinner approximately three times a week each. Choose lean cuts of beef or pork one or two times a week.

HERE'S WHY The omega-3 fatty acids in fish act like a sort of biological antifreeze, keeping arteries from clogging. Skinless chicken, especially white meat, is another good low-fat choice. Loin cuts of beef and pork can be almost as low in fat as chicken, but beware of the fat in heavily marbled cuts of red meat or regular ground beef. It's saturated, which means that it raises your cholesterol and fat deposits in your arteries. By switching from a typical burger at lunch to one made from lean ground beef or ground turkey, you'll save between 5 to 10 grams of saturated fat—about a third of a day's worth —with one meal.

HERE'S HOW

- Choose fish three times a week: a tuna sandwich for lunch, and broiled salmon or pasta with clams for dinner.
- Check the recipes in the back of this book for new ways to prepare fish.
- At restaurants, order a grilled chicken sandwich (hold the fries) or if you must have a burger, order the smallest one on the menu, without cheese, bacon, or special sauce.

- **STEP 3:** Eat no more than 2 ounces of regular (full-fat) cheese a week.

HERE'S WHY Smoking raises your blood cholesterol level, and if yours is already high, cutting back on cheese when you quit is a good way to begin to bring it back to normal. That's because cheese (along with beef and whole milk) is one of the top three sources of saturated fat in the diet. Like smoking, saturated fat is a culprit in raising blood cholesterol.

Many people eat too much cheese because it's convenient and it's a component of other favorite convenience foods, especially pizza. But too much cheese offsets all the positive changes people have made in their diets, such as eating more lean meats, grains, and vegetables. Each ounce of full-fat cheese, such as cheddar, Swiss, or jarlsburg, contains 4 to 6 grams of saturated fat. An ounce is just 1⅓ slices of American, ¼ cup shredded cheese, or a 1½-inch cube of hard cheese—an amount you'd likely get in one medium-sized slice of pizza.

HERE'S HOW

- Cheese can fit into a low-fat diet if eaten in *small* amounts as the *sole* source of protein at lunch or dinner. Avoid adding cheese to sandwiches, burgers, salads, and other favorites that already contain protein.
- Order pizza with half the usual cheese and opt for low-fat protein toppings of chicken or shrimp rather than pepperoni or sausage.

Don't forget to ask for sliced tomatoes, mushrooms, broccoli, bell peppers, and onions.

- Try different reduced-fat or fat-free cheeses until you find a brand you like.
- Since Americans eat more mozzarella than any other cheese, try using light (half the fat of part-skim) or part-skim (1 gram of saturated fat less per ounce than regular) varieties.
- Use a small amount of a strong-flavored cheese, such as Parmesan, instead of a larger amount of a milder cheese. Freshly grated Parmesan has more pungent flavor than the canned variety, which makes it easier to use less for the same flavor.

- **STEP 4:** Choose a sandwich for lunch, but switch from high-fat to lower-fat sandwich fillings and condiments, and watch the size of your sandwich.

HERE'S WHY Processed meats, such as hot dogs, sausage, bologna, and bacon, are high in saturated fat as well as sodium. A B.L.T. from a typical deli has 840 calories, more than half a day's fat (40 grams) and saturated fat (12 grams), and nearly a whole day's sodium (2,200 mg).

A sandwich made at home—two slices of bread, 3 to 4 ounces of protein, mustard, lettuce, and tomato—is approximately 400 to 500 calories, or about 100 calories per ounce. If you order the same sandwich at a deli or restaurant, it might come with more bread, more filling, and more fattening additions such as mayonnaise or Russian dressing. An 8- to 10-ounce restaurant sandwich probably contains 800 to 1,000 calories. Eat half and share the other half with a friend, or save it for the next day's lunch.

HERE'S HOW
- When making sandwiches at home, begin with good whole-grain bread (around 100 calories and at least 2 grams of fiber per slice).
- Buy deli-fresh turkey or lean ham or beef, and keep sandwich fillings to 3 ounces or less.
- Buy low-fat or fat-free bologna or hot dogs. Hormel's Light and Lean hot dogs contain only 1 gram of fat each. Check those made by Healthy Choice and Oscar Mayer as well.

- Try low-fat sausage such as Morningstar Farms Grillers.
- Use fat-free or low-fat condiments such as mustard, reduced-fat mayonnaise, salsas, and some chutneys.
- Fill sandwiches with healthy veggies, such as lettuce, tomato, and onion, or other vegetables grilled or roasted with little to no oil. This will add bulk and fiber to your sandwich, making you feel fuller.

- **STEP 5:** Eat at least three servings of vegetables at lunch or dinner, and two servings of fruit as snacks each day.

HERE'S WHY Smoking depletes the body of several vitamins found in fruits and vegetables, including vitamins A and C, and folic acid. Some of these vitamins may help prevent heart disease and stroke, along with cancers of the lung, colon, stomach, esophagus, mouth, throat, and possibly the bladder and cervix. Eating more fruits and vegetables will help bring your vitamin levels back up, which is especially important since smokers tend to be at higher risk for many of these conditions.

Of course, it's fine to eat vegetables as snacks and fruit during meals, but the more typical way to get your vitamin quota is to eat two or three pieces of fruit as snacks throughout the day, and have a good portion of vegetables at dinner (and lunch, if possible). This way, in addition to getting an infusion of vitamins, minerals, and fiber, you are likely to be replacing less healthy vending machine snacks, such as chips and candy, with bananas, oranges, and apples. At dinner, vegetables may help control the number of calories consumed by increasing satiety before you've eaten too many pasta, rice, or potato servings.

HERE'S HOW
- The United States Department of Agriculture (U.S.D.A.) Food Guide Pyramid defines a single serving as ½ cup of fruit or vegetables. These portions, which work out to about ½ banana or a small serving of broccoli, are probably less than you're likely to eat in one sitting—so it's easy to reach your goal.

- Carry fruit at all times. An apple, orange, or banana is easy to take with you wherever you go, and not always easy to find once you're away from your home.
- Freeze overripe bananas to use as a smoothie base. Then toss in frozen strawberries, mangos, and blueberries for those times when you run out of fresh fruit. You'll find a great shake recipe on page 161.
- Add dried fruits such as raisins, apricots, or cranberries to oatmeal, or use these fruits as dry cereal toppings. They also make excellent transportable snacks.
- Rely on fresh fruits rather than fruit juices. Natural fruits are more filling, higher in fiber, and lower in calories than their juice counterparts. Consider that it takes three apples to make 1 cup of apple juice.
- Make salads from romaine lettuce or spinach rather than iceberg lettuce. The greener the greens, the more nutrients they contain. Rather than relying solely on salads for your vegetable, add a vegetable on the side, or skip the salad and have a hefty serving (1 to 2 cups) of broccoli, green beans, or carrots.
- Don't be afraid to add a smidgen of olive or canola oil if you're bored with plain steamed vegetables. Stir-fry or sauté broccoli with a little onion, garlic, and oil. Add a splash of water or chicken broth to steam it as needed. Season with low-sodium soy sauce, anchovy paste, basil, or rosemary. Check the recipes on pages 247 to 260 for more savory tips.

- **STEP 6:** Switch from whole or 2% fat dairy products to nonfat or 1% (skim).

HERE'S WHY Full-fat dairy products such as ice cream, whole milk, and whole-milk yogurt add a significant amount of saturated fat and cholesterol to the diet. The reduced-fat versions offer the same calcium benefits, sometimes a bit better, without the high levels of saturated fat.

- Switch to skim milk rather than whole milk and save 5 grams of saturated fat per serving.
- Instead of premium full-fat ice creams (14 grams of fat per ½ cup), try low-fat ice cream or frozen yogurt (about 3 grams per ½ cup), a savings of 11 grams of fat. Sorbet or fruit ice, although not a dairy product, is also a refreshing fat-free dessert option.
- Fat-free or low-fat yogurt—or fat-free sour cream—makes a fine substitute for regular sour cream in many dishes. Sometimes too just a small dollop of the real thing makes a big difference in flavor and texture. For dips, try mixing a little regular sour cream with low-fat cottage cheese, fat-free yogurt, or fat-free mayonnaise.

- **STEP 7:** Make at least 50 percent of your grain choices whole grains.

HERE'S WHY Smokers tend to have lower blood levels of vitamin B_6, and an easy way for new ex-smokers to raise those levels is to increase the amount of whole grains they eat. Whole grains also provide more fiber, zinc, copper, manganese, potassium, and other B vitamins than refined grain products, nutrients that can help lower the risk of heart disease, diverticulosis, and cancer. The American Cancer Society recommends 20 to 30 grams of fiber a day; most Americans get just 10 to 12 grams. Insoluble fiber (in whole-grain wheat products) helps keep your bowels regular, and soluble fiber (in oatmeal, dried beans, and legumes such as refried pinto beans, black beans, lentils, split peas) helps lower cholesterol levels. The final bonus: Whole grains are usually more filling than an equal amount of refined grains, which means you eat less and take in fewer calories.

HERE'S HOW

- Start your day with a bowl of oatmeal, or check the breakfast recipes on pages 153 to 165 for other ways to incorporate oats into your diet. If you prefer cold cereal, choose one that's whole grain with at least 2 to 6 grams of fiber per serving. Good choices are Fiber One, Shredded Wheat, Nutri-Grain, Total, Cheerios, and bran flakes.

- Find a good whole-grain bread that you like and stick with it for sandwiches and toast. Look for a brand that offers at least 2 grams of fiber per slice.
- Choose whole-grain crackers such as Wheatsworth, Rye Crisp, or Triscuits.
- Consider changing to brown rice and whole-wheat pasta.

- **STEP 8:** Replace butter or margarine with olive oil or canola oil.

HERE'S WHY Butter is a major source of fat and saturated fat in the average person's diet. And margarine, although it contains less saturated fat than butter, contains trans fat, which raises cholesterol levels. By using a tablespoon of canola oil or olive oil in place of butter, you'll save 7 grams of saturated fat; plus, olive oil contains mostly monounsaturated fats which, unlike polyunsaturated fats, lower LDL cholesterol (the bad one) while protecting HDL cholesterol (the good one). If you're replacing margarine, you'll save approximately 1 gram of saturated fat per tablespoon.

HERE'S HOW
- Lightly dip bread in olive oil seasoned with garlic, but be careful not to overdo it. A tablespoon of olive oil is about 100 calories, and that should suffice. When grilling bread, spray the slice with vegetable oil spray before placing it in a hot skillet or under the broiler.
- To top toast or muffins, skip the fat altogether and spread with all-fruit jam or jelly, a little honey, or light cream cheese. If you must use margarine, use the lower-fat tub margarine like Smart Beat, Fleischmann's Lower Fat, or Promise Ultra. If you're stuck on butter, make it a light whipped brand and use sparingly. Because of the air whipped in, you'll save over 3 grams of fat per tablespoon, 2 grams of which are saturated.
- For cooking and baking, use olive oil or canola oil. Oils can add a distinct flavor and richness to foods; just keep the amount to 1 teaspoon per serving.

• **STEP 9:** Switch from regular soda pop to water, nonfat milk, diet soda, or a low-calorie drink mix, such as Crystal Light.

HERE'S WHY If you want to avoid weight gain, don't waste 150 calories—equal to 10 teaspoons of sugar or two slices of bread—on a 12-ounce can of soda pop. The best choice is plain old water. Water is not only essential for all body processes, but an integral part of an overall healthy diet as well. Drinking enough water can also help new ex-smokers fight off the sense of fatigue caused by low-grade dehydration, which they frequently experience during the first few weeks without cigarettes.

HERE'S HOW
- Switch to diet soft drinks for zero calories (but limit them to two per day so you don't introduce too many artificial sweeteners into your diet), or nonfat milk for calories chock-full of protein, calcium, and B vitamins.
- Drink 6 to 8 glasses of water a day.
- If you want to drink fruit juice instead of soda pop, which contain about the same amount of calories, remember that fruit juice also provides lots of vitamins and minerals. Dilute your juice with club soda to lower calories per serving, and add a twist of lemon for extra punch.

• **STEP 10:** Take a vitamin-mineral supplement.

HERE'S WHY Countless national nutrition surveys report that Americans do not consume adequate, let alone optimal, amounts of necessary vitamins and minerals. If you've been a smoker, you're even more likely to fall short of one or more essential nutrients, such as vitamins B_6, A, C, and folic acid, particularly if you consume less than 2,500 calories a day. A vitamin-mineral supplement can provide you with good nutritional insurance during those crucial early weeks of smoking cessation when your body breaks its nicotine addiction and your new healthy diet begins to supply you with all the vitamins and minerals you need. But avoid thinking that if a little is good, more is better, since some vitamins and minerals are toxic in large doses. Megadoses of vitamins is a form of self-medication and any extended vitamin therapy should be monitored by a physician schooled in nutritional science.

Getting Your Antioxidants

Cigarette smoke releases free radicals in the lungs, which can damage the DNA in cells. This puts smokers at an increased risk for lung cancer, so it's especially important for them to get plenty of antioxidants, which help neutralize free radicals. Antioxidants include vitamins C, E, and beta carotene.

• **VITAMIN C:** Smoking apparently causes vitamin C to break down in the body faster than normal, which may explain why vitamin C levels in the blood of smokers are 30 to 50 percent lower than in nonsmokers. In fact, the National Academy of Sciences officially increased the Recommended Dietary Allowance (RDA) of vitamin C for those who smoke. Vitamin C is required for fighting infections since it is used to maintain white blood cells. The best food sources are citrus fruits, broccoli, strawberries, cantaloupe, and bell peppers.

• **VITAMIN E:** This antioxidant blocks the oxidation of beta carotene and protects the lung tissue from the harmful oxidants found in cigarette smoke. Research shows that smokers have less vitamin E in their lung fluid than nonsmokers, which may mean that vitamin E is used up combating smoke oxidants. The good news for new ex-smokers is that the combination of increasing vitamin E intake and decreasing smoke inhaled will help bring the level of vitamin E in the lungs closer to normal. Good sources of vitamin E include nuts, seeds, oils (especially cold-pressed), avocado, broccoli, and whole-grain breads and cereals (which contain the wheat germ portion of the wheat kernel where vitamin E is found).

• **BETA CAROTENE:** Although we hear mainly of its antioxidant properties, beta carotene's primary function is to be converted into vitamin A, which helps maintain the soundness of tissues in the body, including the lining of the lungs and bronchial passages. High levels of beta carotene in the blood protect against some forms of cancer, including lung cancer. Since vitamin A is broken down faster than normal in the body of a smoker, carcinogens may be able to invade the lung tissue more readily. Good sources of vitamin A or its precursor, beta carotene, which converts to the active form of vitamin A while in the body, are dark green and orange vegetables and fruits such as broccoli, asparagus, sweet potatoes, yams, apricots, and cantaloupe.

• **SELENIUM:** Selenium is a trace mineral, required by the body in very small amounts. Like vitamins C, E, and beta carotene, it's an antioxidant that helps protect the cells of the respiratory tract from damage by oxidants in cigarette smoke. In addition, selenium detoxifies heavy metals such as mercury and cadmium that are present in cigarette smoke. Since selenium is potentially toxic, avoid more than 200 mcg per day from foods you eat and supplement sources. Foods rich in selenium include seafood, beef, pork, lamb, chicken, organ meats, broccoli, cabbage, onions, mushrooms, and grains.

• **VITAMIN B$_{12}$:** Other vitamins especially important for smokers and new ex-smokers are the B-complex vitamins. Various substances in tobacco smoke appear to interfere with the body's ability to absorb certain vitamins. Nitrous oxide in cigarette smoke, for example, breaks down vitamin B$_{12}$, resulting in its excretion through the urine and a depleted level in most smokers. Vitamin B$_{12}$ helps the stress response in the body. Good sources include red meats, dairy products, and eggs. For vegetarians, choose miso, tempeh, and yogurt with active cultures.

• **FOLIC ACID:** Folic acid is partially inactivated by smoking. Involved in red blood cell formation, folic acid is also known to prevent certain birth defects, making it important for pregnant women. Some good sources are spinach and other leafy greens such as kale, collard greens and romaine lettuce, orange juice, kidney beans, avocado, asparagus, and beets.

• **CALCIUM:** Smoking has been found to increase the risk of osteoporosis, so smokers and new ex-smokers need to make sure they get plenty of calcium in their diets. But boosting calcium intake alone will not protect you from osteoporosis. In addition, you can prevent bone loss by getting lots of weight-bearing exercise, such as walking. Vitamin D and phosphorous help the body absorb calcium, and estrogen helps prevent bone loss.

Another function of calcium is to regulate blood pressure, which in smokers can be elevated by 10 to 15 percent. The carbon monoxide in smoke displaces some of the oxygen that red blood cells normally transport throughout the body. Since there is less oxygen in the blood, the heart must beat harder and faster to deliver enough oxygen to the various organs, thus increasing blood pressure after each cigarette. Good sources of calcium include dairy products, fortified soy products, fortified orange juice, fortified rice, legumes, dark green vegetables, broccoli, nuts and seeds, figs, and black-strap molasses.

Selecting Your Supplement

• **VITAMINS:** Choose a multiple vitamin-mineral preparation rather than several single supplements. That way, you'll have fewer pills to swallow and be spending less money than you would buying all those vitamins in separate pills. Select a supplement that provides approximately 100 to 300 percent of the U.S. RDA for the following vitamins: fat-soluble vitamins A (preferably beta carotene) and E; and water-soluble vitamins C, B_1, B_2, niacin, B_6, B_{12}, folic acid, pantothenic acid, and biotin. Vitamin D can be toxic in large amounts, so total intake from fortified foods such as milk, cereals, and supplements should be no more than 200 percent of the U.S. RDA, or 400 IU. The following single supplements are recommended: vitamin C (up to 1,000 mg), vitamin E (up to 400 IU), and beta carotene (up to 25,000 IU).

• **MINERALS:** Choose a supplement that provides the following minerals in these approximate amounts: chromium (50 to 200 mcg), manganese (2.5 to 5.0 mg), and selenium (50 to 200 mcg). It should also contain calcium, copper, iron, magnesium, and zinc. Most multiples, however, do not contain adequate amounts of calcium since it tends to make the pill too large to swallow. Consider taking an additional single supplement of calcium. (Men need 800 mg; women need 800 mg and 1,200 mg after menopause.)

Other substances found in foods, but not in supplements, protect against disease and improve health—making a strong case for food as your best source of vitamins and minerals. Here's a rundown of some of the most important ones. The menu plans and recipes found on pages 80 to 97 suggest ways to incorporate these substances into your diet.

• **INDOLES:** Found in the cabbage family of vegetables, including broccoli, cauliflower, and cabbage; may boost production of enzymes that eliminate cancer-causing chemicals.

• **BETA GLUCAN:** Fiber found in oats, carrots, and dried cooked beans and peas; helps lower cholesterol.

- **RESVERATROL:**   Antioxidant found in grapes and red wine that may prevent free radical damage, which damages linings of arteries.
- **GREEN TEA:**   Contains potent antioxidant chemicals known as polyphenols, which may be even more powerful disease fighters than vitamin E or C.
- **LYCOPENE:**   The pigment in tomatoes; when cooked, may help protect against developing cancer.
- **ALLYL SULFIDES:**   Found in garlic, chives, and onions; may help the body destroy cancer-causing chemicals more safely. No need to cook these foods, just cut them up and let them sit for at least 10 minutes for maximum effectiveness.

FOR THOSE WITH SPECIAL NEEDS

Smoking raises blood pressure temporarily with every cigarette. Exercise conversely reduces blood pressure. If you still have a problem with high blood pressure, cutting back on sodium can help, particularly if you're salt sensitive. Not everyone with high blood pressure responds to changes in dietary sodium; there's really no way of determining who will and who won't. But it's wise to keep sodium intake in check even if you *don't* have a problem with your blood pressure. The goal is to keep sodium to about 2,000 milligrams a day. Check labels and limit foods that contain more than 480 milligrams of sodium per serving—that's the government's cut-off point when it comes to labeling foods as "healthy."

HERE'S HOW
- Avoid or limit processed foods such as canned soups, pizza (especially with salty toppings like sausage or anchovies), frozen dinners, lunch meats, hot dogs, and ham.
- Avoid adding excessive salt from the salt shaker. One teaspoon of salt contains 2,400 milligrams of sodium.

MAKING THE PLAN WORK
MEANS LEARNING TO EAT
THE RIGHT AMOUNTS

Although eating wholesome, nutritious foods can help keep you healthy, the trick to losing weight is to eat such foods in the right amounts. Overeating healthy food also leads to weight gain so it's important to eat the correct number of calories.

Portion size is also the key when you're treating yourself to higher-fat indulgences. For example, if absentminded snacking on nuts means you eat a quarter of a standard can, you'll have munched on about 40 grams of fat—almost a day's worth for most people! On the other hand, a half ounce, the size of an airplane bag of peanuts, is a satisfying, crunchy snack with B-vitamins, zinc, and fiber, and contains only 8 grams of fat, mostly the good monounsaturated kind.

If you're just quitting smoking, use the checklist below as your starting point. If you quit some time ago and are trying to lose the weight that you gained, you're ready for the Personal Nutrition Management Plan in Chapter 5, which is more specific about portion size.

USE THE CHECKLIST

The following checklist specifies the minimum and maximum number of foods you need every day. To lose weight, cut back on the extras. Limit your daily intake of milk and legumes/meat to the recommended two to three servings each, and grains (preferably whole grains) to six servings. Make up the rest of your calorie allotment with vegetables, fruits, and additional servings of whole grains. Copy this checklist to keep yourself on track daily.

FOOD SERVING CHECKLIST

FOOD	SERVING SIZE	GOAL	SERVINGS CONSUMED	MET GOAL?	
GRAINS/BREAD	½ cup cooked grains 1 slice bread ½ bagel ½ English muffin	6–11	_____	Yes	No
	(Of these grains, how many were whole grain?)	4–11	_____	Yes	No
VEGETABLES	1 piece ½ cup cooked 1 cup raw or frozen	3–5+	_____	Yes	No
	(Of those veggies, how many were dark green?)	1–2+	_____	Yes	No
FRUITS	1 piece ½ cup canned 1 cup raw	2–4	_____	Yes	No
	(Of those fruits, how many were citrus or high in vitamin C?)	1–2+	_____	Yes	No
MILK (low-fat/nonfat)	8 ounces milk/yogurt 1 ounce low-fat cheese	2–3	_____	Yes	No
LEGUMES/MEAT (extra lean)/POULTRY (skinless)/FISH	3 ounces meat, chicken, or fish 1 cup beans/peas	2–3	_____	Yes	No
WATER	1 8-ounce glass	6–8+	_____	Yes	No
EXTRAS (sweets, oils, fats, alcohol)	1 tablespoon oil/fat 1 small dessert 2 tablespoons sugar 8 ounces soda (regular) 1 alcoholic beverage	0–3	_____	Yes	No

CHAPTER 5
The Personal Nutrition Management Plan with Menu Plans

Congratulations! Now that you've reached this part of the book, you're probably already following the eating guidelines set out in Chapter 4 and have made the commitment to quit cigarettes for good. The next step involves more structure than you may be used to, but it's worth it. The goal is to learn to eat healthful foods in the right amounts and in the right balance. To reach that goal, the Personal Nutrition Management Plan, which I developed and have used successfully with hundreds of clients, provides you with all the dietary tools you need to maintain your weight during the first few weeks of smoking cessation—and beyond. But first a word about the latest diet trends.

WHAT ABOUT ALL THOSE POPULAR DIETS?

Over the years, you may have tried the Atkins Diet, the Drinking Man's Diet, vegetarian diets, liquid protein diets, counting fat grams, or even fasting. You may have adopted the diet of marathon runners and triathletes, even if the most exercise you got was walking from the front door to the car door each morning. Or you might have embarked on one of those low-fat, high-complex carbohydrate diets that were popular in the late 1980s—which were very appealing to those of us who loved bread and pasta. But if you thought that no fat meant no calories, you probably learned pretty quickly that too many carbohydrates translated into too many calories, and that led directly to weight gain instead of weight loss. Without proper boundaries, there was a tendency to rely on fat-free salad dressings, fat-free muffins, and fat-free desserts—foods that were missing fat but high in carbohydrates—instead of a structured, healthy, balanced diet.

Now the hot diet advice is to cut out carbohydrates, add more protein, and not worry too much about fatty foods. The appeal of this high-protein regime is fast weight loss, and the weight loss at the beginning of this type of diet is often dramatic. But it's largely just water, resulting from the liberation of stored water due to severe carbohydrate restriction. Diet gurus will have you believe that there are many hormonal and scientific reasons for their low-carbohydrate diets to work. But the real reason is much simpler and not quite as revolutionary as the gurus claim: Calories are reduced.

And calories do count. It's an old message that's been preached before. But it was probably forgotten by a lot of people in the past who carbo-loaded and sought out low-fat and nonfat foods almost exclusively. Many dieters clearly lost sight of the calories contained in the foods they were eating, especially if the label on the package read "low-fat" or "nonfat." When fat is removed, sugar or other carbohydrate-based sweeteners are often added, boosting the calorie level so that nonfat products can contain even more calories than low-fat foods.

The message of the 1980s—"cut back on fat and eat carbohydrates"— was good. But carbohydrate-craving dieters didn't hear the whole prescription. They ate too much and lost sight of one of the basic weight-loss rules: EAT CONTROLLED PORTIONS. And many ignored the fact that some sort of aerobic exercise was necessary to burn off all that bread and pasta.

So are high-protein diets the answer? Not necessarily. The theme you will hear in the Personal Nutrition Management Plan is the obvious one— moderation. A balanced diet packed with vitamins and minerals, coupled with a regular exercise program to keep you fit, can help you avoid weight gain after you quit smoking. If followed properly, this plan might even help you lose some of the weight you have already gained.

THE PERSONAL NUTRITION MANAGEMENT PLAN

With the Personal Nutrition Management approach, you will not be "dieting." But that doesn't mean you can ignore what you eat.

Moderation means making healthy food choices according to the guidelines outlined in Chapter 4: Eat more fruits and vegetables, breads, and whole grains; go easy on fatty meats, cheese, butter, cream, pastries, and sweets; and eat the right number of calories, based on portions that will keep you within your calorie range (see Step 3, page 53). Whether you're making a food choice at a grocery store, restaurant, or social event, moderation means choosing the healthy alternative. You must eat consciously, paying attention to your level of hunger and fullness (see Step 5, page 55). Minimize inappropriate snacking (see Chapter 8, page 116), and avoid putting any food completely off limits—when the craving strikes, give yourself permission to indulge in small, controlled portions of special foods now and then.

When it comes to quitting smoking, you have to quit completely, and that means NO TOBACCO. But when it comes to weight loss, perfection isn't the goal. Keep your efforts in perspective to help you through the tough times. A minor eating indiscretion won't affect your weight or your health—it's what you do on a routine basis that counts. Trying to be a "perfect" dieter can in fact sabotage your goal and make you abandon all your efforts. For example, after a slip-up you might say to yourself, "I ate too much food at the barbecue on Friday night. I blew it and I might as well keep eating badly this weekend. I'll start again on Monday." Instead, focus on your good eating habits and get back to them at the next meal, whether that's breakfast, lunch, or dinner. You'll read more about how to overcome self-defeating thoughts on page 98.

Some people don't like the idea of moderation. They're convinced it couldn't possibly work for them because they were only able to lose weight in the past by going on a restrictive diet. That may work for the short term, but these people soon find themselves on a seesaw of stringent dieting followed by out-of-control eating. Successful implementation of the principle of moderation will lead you to feel in control and more self-confident about your ability to maintain a healthy diet. It's the guiding rule for life-long success with weight management. Start now.

Here are four basic steps designed to help you achieve success.

STEP 1: SET REALISTIC WEIGHT GOALS.

Once you've made your commitment to moderation, the next step is to set *realistic* weight goals. That doesn't mean setting goals that will let you achieve society's ideal of thinness. Instead, take into consideration the body shape you've inherited: Are you a pear or an apple, tall or short? Your goal should be to do the best with what you have so that you can be as vital and physically fit as possible.

Let health and fitness without tobacco be the focus of your life. Begin with a long-term goal. Perhaps you've been carrying around extra weight for some time, and want to get back to what you weighed in the past. Maybe it was what you weighed in high school or at your 10th reunion, or maybe it was the weight you were that summer a couple of years ago when you felt great about yourself. Whatever it is, make sure that your goal is healthy and realistic rather than ideal and unlikely. Be open to revising your weight goal up or down as you progress. You must also have a temporary goal, one that's no more than 10 pounds below your present weight.

Finally, when setting your goal, consider your body composition. Focusing on what the scale says alone is often misleading. The scale measures overall body mass and does not take into account the proportion of fat to lean body mass.

How Fast Will I Lose Weight?

Many eager dieters expect to lose a pound or two a week. They often do the first few weeks, but it's only from water loss that occurs when they eat less food. A pound or two a month is a much more realistic goal for the long term. Your rate of weight loss depends both on your height and how much weight you have to lose. Generally, a small woman loses weight at a slower rate than a tall man, simply because she has less muscle mass and therefore burns fewer calories, so it's harder for her to create a calorie deficit.

When Should I Start?

If you've just quit smoking or are about to quit, don't pressure yourself too much about losing weight. It will distract you from the real task of learning to live without tobacco. In fact, the Smoking Cessation Clinical Practice

Guidelines, published by the Agency for Health Care Policy and Research in 1996, suggest that attempting to go on a restrictive diet in the early stages of quitting may actually undermine your efforts. If you've made it through the first tough week or two of nicotine withdrawal, you have passed the most important marker for success. Reaching the 12-week point, however, means you've arrived at a much lower risk for relapsing. At that point you might begin following the recommendations set out in the PNM plan. Only when you're truly past the riskiest point for relapse—those first 12 weeks—will you feel comfortable enough to redirect your energies and focus on long-term weight loss. But keep in mind that your first priority is to "stay quit."

STEP 2: ESTIMATE YOUR CALORIE NEED.

When following the food recommendations in Chapter 4, remember to stay within your calorie goals, or slightly below them when adjusted for exercise and the presumed 200-calorie decrease you may experience when you quit smoking. But just what are your calorie needs? The amount of calories your body needs is determined by adding your basal metabolic rate (BMR), or calories burned at rest, to the energy required to digest food and engage in daily activity. According to the National Research Council, average daily calorie requirements range from 2,400 calories per day for older men to 3,000 for younger men, and 1,800 calories per day for older women to 2,100 calories for younger women.

Choose your beginning calorie goal according to the following formula: First, add a "0" at the end of your present weight in pounds. Then if you're a woman, add your weight again to that figure; if you're a man, double your weight and add it to that figure. This will give you an estimate of your BMR. Take 30 percent of that number for an estimate of your daily activity needs. Now add the two numbers together to get an estimate of your total daily energy need. For example, a 130-pound younger woman would add 1,300 to 130 for an estimated BMR of 1,430, and then add 30 percent of that figure, or approximately 430, for a total estimated daily calorie need of 1,860. This is a good starting place, but keep in mind that you must also discover what level of calories will produce—and maintain—the weight results you want.

How Low Can I Go?

Don't sabotage your weight-loss efforts by adopting a level of calories that's just too low. If you are tempted to eat too few calories, remember that even if you're able to stay with the regimen (which, fortunately, you probably won't be), you'd likely lose as much lean body mass (i.e., muscle) and water as fat. In addition, your metabolic rate could decrease by as much as 20 percent—so that when you returned to your usual calorie intake, you'd *gain* weight at the same calorie level you formerly maintained.

Too few calories also means that you'd be hungry all the time, you wouldn't get enough nutrients, and you'd lack the energy for exercise. The typical restrictive diet won't get you results, but it can result in fatigue, depression, guilt, anger toward yourself, and lower self-esteem. Be satisfied with a steady, slow weight loss. Think of two pounds a month as 24 pounds a year. Make sure you eat enough food so you don't feel deprived, and develop a plan you can live with over the long term.

How Do Calories Relate to Pounds?

The idea that you can calculate your daily calorie need, and then cut out a predetermined number of calories to produce a given weight loss shouldn't be taken too literally. For example, if you maintain your weight at 1,800 calories and then reduce your food intake by 500 calories per day, you should theoretically lose one pound of fat in a week (500 calories × 7 days = 3500 calories = a pound of fat). In fact, you'd probably lose more than one pound initially, and then less and less. Over time your metabolism would adapt and slow down to protect your body from what it perceives as "starvation."

Although it's a good idea to have a daily calorie goal, allow yourself to eat more if you're hungry. As long as you're responding to stomach hunger (see the chart on page 76), you won't have any problem. On the other hand, if you find that you're too full after a meal or not hungry at mealtimes, try to eat less the rest of the day. The final verdict will lie in your own weight fluctuation. If you keep a record of how much you eat and get on the scale once a week, you'll have a pretty accurate idea of how to adjust your food intake. If you're having trouble, see a registered dietitian; he or she can help you estimate your calorie needs and work out a sensible food plan.

Learning complicated, detailed nutritional parameters can put you at risk for developing the "dieter's mentality," which can be self-defeating. But if you like details, you may find it helpful to refer to the chart in the appendix for specifics about carbohydrate and fat goals. Just remember to use the numbers as rough guidelines and not final arbiters.

Can Too Much Restriction Be Bad for Me?

As discussed in Chapter 3, the appetite control center in the brain kicks in when we restrict calories too severely. If you're very rigid about which foods you allow yourself to eat, you're likely to overeat when you have a glass of wine, get distracted, or feel upset. "Giving in" to a food you've labeled as "forbidden" can start a temporary downward spiral in which you can't get enough. Putting a particular food off limits generally makes you crave it all the more.

One of my clients, Susan, categorized all foods as "good" or "bad." Whenever she ate a bad food, she'd immediately feel so guilty that she was unable to enjoy it. Instead she'd bolt down the offending food when no one was looking just as fast as she could, almost as if she could deny to herself that she was actually eating it. She said she felt deprived for so long that the moment she took one bite, she lost all self-control. But once she stopped labeling food as good or bad, and gave herself permission to eat a cookie now and then, she began to regain her self-control.

Take your time. Enjoy an indulgence. Remember that the taste of a sweet treat is most appreciated in the first few bites. Savor it and you'll be satisfied with less. Losing weight and being fit does not mean giving up all your treats all the time. In fact, eating foods you love keeps you from thinking you're "on" a diet, which is just another label and adds more pressure. Focus on making wise food choices *most* of the time. For more information on handling those "trigger foods," see page 122.

STEP 3: WRITE IT DOWN.

Once you've determined your fat and calorie goals, keep a record of what you eat, how many calories the food contains, and the number of calories you expend from exercise. Although it's tedious, counting calories can be an eye-opening exercise. (You won't need to count fat grams if you follow the guidelines in Chapter 4 and/or the menu plans, since they're calculated to keep you in the optimal range of 20 to 30 percent of total calories as fat.)

How Long Should I Keep my Food/Exercise Journal?

Try it for at least a week or two, until you have a sense of the calorie range you're in. Keep it up if you find that it's helpful—many people do. Monitoring your food intake and exercise levels allows you to make more choices than you would if you followed a rigid food plan. If you don't count calories, you can fool yourself into thinking that you're cutting back when you're not. Use the calorie counter in the back of the book, or purchase a more complete list of food values at your local bookstore.

Make copies of the chart on page 74 to help you monitor your progress.

What About Problem Areas?

In your journal, make a note of problem areas such as:

- Situations that lead to overeating—e.g., parties, restaurants, Mom's house.
- Emotions that trigger excessive eating—e.g., anger, stress, boredom.
- Times when you eat too fast.
- Instances when you feel the need to clean your plate rather than stop eating when you're comfortably full.
- Periods of unconscious eating—being unaware of the hand-to-mouth activity that happens when you're watching a movie, sitting at your desk, driving in your car, etc.

Just as you analyzed your smoking style, by becoming aware of your eating style you can understand where your problems lie and work on the areas you want to change. Concentrate on the challenges that will have the most impact, and then fine-tune the other areas.

FOOD JOURNAL

NAME: _____

DATE: _____

DAY: M T W Th F Sa Su

TIME	FOOD AND QUANTITY	CALORIES	DP	B/MP	F/V	G	O	HUNGER SCALE 0 1 2 3 4 5 6 7 8 9 10	MOOD, THOUGHTS AND/OR FEELINGS
TOTALS									
RECOMMENDED								0 = Empty 5 = Neutral 10 = Stuffed	Graph hunger level from start to end of meal.

EXERCISE: _____

DP = Dairy Protein
B/MP = Bean/Meat Protein
F/V = Fruit/Vegetable
G = Grain
0 = Others

STEP 4: LEARN TO EAT WHEN YOU'RE HUNGRY AND STOP WHEN YOU'RE FULL.

If counting calories feels too much like "dieting," then relief is in sight. Although the Personal Nutrition Management Plan suggests monitoring calorie levels as a starting point, it's up to you to determine when and how much to eat. The way to do this is by relying on your body's own feelings of hunger and fullness—only you know how much food you need. Be honest with your physical sensations, in the same way that you try to be honest with your emotions. Learn to listen to what your body says.

If you're hungry—that stomach-growling, empty feeling—you know it's time to eat. No one ever became overweight by responding to genuine hunger cues. This is different, of course, than eating because the clock says it's dinnertime, or because you're sitting with friends in a restaurant, or you've gone out with the gang after work for drinks and chips and dip. Remember to respond *only* to real hunger and to ignore false urges, just as you learned to ignore nicotine cravings when you quit smoking.

Similarly, you must recognize when you have had enough to eat and *stop eating*. "Having enough" means feeling the sensation of fullness in your belly—*before* you get to the point of feeling stuffed. As discussed on page 117, we tend to eat about two pounds of food each day, and choosing minimally processed foods—i.e., plenty of fruits, vegetables, and whole grains—will help you feel satisfied. You must respond to the body's needs for carbohydrates, protein, and fat, but you must also stay aware of other physical cues. Thus you don't always have to clean your plate; your body might tell you that you feel full after you've eaten two-thirds of your portion.

How Can I Help Myself to Stop?

Memorize the following statements and say them aloud whether you're dining with someone or alone. They will help you stop eating when you're full.

"I'm so full, I couldn't eat another bite."

"It was delicious but I'm absolutely stuffed. No thank you."

"Thank you, but I'll pass on dessert."

But What If It's Emotional?

The following scale provides you with signposts to help you listen to your body.

10—absolutely, positively, lie-on-the-floor stuffed
9—so full that I am starting to hurt
8—very full and bloated
7—starting to feel uncomfortable
6—slightly too full
5—perfectly comfortable
4—experiencing first signals that it's time to eat
3—experiencing strong signals to eat
2—very hungry, irritable
1—extremely hungry, dizzy

If you are at level 5 or higher, you are not hungry and your body and brain don't need anything. If you are craving something, it's not biological—it's emotional. If you are at level 3 or 4, your body is telling you specifically that it needs food. Give yourself permission to eat, but remember to control your portions and stop when you're full.

The best way to manage your weight is to focus on healthy eating behaviors that help you lose weight slowly and steadily; behaviors that train you to adopt a healthy food plan that's so simple it becomes a way of life. With that in mind, the following menus will guide you through the first three weeks to make sure you're in the ballpark of the nutritional ideal.

WHAT TO EAT ON YOUR QUIT DAY

Whatever path brought you to this day, the Personal Nutrition Management Plan has a special one-day eating plan to make it easier for you to get started on kicking the habit. It's a day to treat yourself, because you're doing something that's very hard on so many levels: physical, psychological, habitual, and emotional. Be especially nice to yourself this day and know that you just might be doing your body the biggest favor in the world.

Wash all your ashtrays and put them away. Throw out all cigarettes. You might even want to do a load of laundry to get the smoky smell out of your clothes. Try to avoid the things that go well with cigarettes or trigger smoking, such as coffee, beer, or even talking on the phone. Read through this section and have the food suggestions ready in the morning. When you wake up, know that this nurturing one-day food plan will help you begin your new nonsmoking life.

Breakfast
Oatmeal with Brown Sugar, Sliced Banana, and Milk
or
Two Eggs Prepared As You Like Them with 2 Slices Toast, each with
    1 teaspoon Butter or Margarine, and 4 ounces Juice

Morning Snack
Apple with Peanut Butter
or
Orange with String Cheese

Lunch
Sandwich of Your Choice
Cookie or small-sized dessert
Milk

Afternoon Snack
Frozen Yogurt with Fruits and Nuts
or
Popsicles with 1 Box Animal Crackers

Dinner
Spaghetti with Meatballs
Green Salad
Garlic Toast

(It's best to avoid alcohol the first week or two as it can impair the decision for tobacco abstinence.)

Dessert
Once you've made it all the way to the evening of your first nonsmoking day, treat yourself to a scoop of your favorite ice cream.

GENERAL RULES—FOR THIS DAY ONLY

1. Have as many pieces of fruit as you want during the day.

2. Have a bag of trail mix ready (oats, nuts, chocolate, or dried fruit) to munch on throughout the day.

3. Drink lots of liquids—at least 8 glasses of water (or the diet soft drink or low-calorie beverage of your choice) to help your body start to cleanse itself of nicotine.

4. If you feel the urge to smoke coming on, eat one of the above mentioned snacks, take a walk, or call a friend. Breathe deeply and wait a few minutes; the urge will pass whether you smoke or not.

END OF DAY RITUAL

At the close of the day, after you've had your ice cream and maybe one final piece of fruit, take a hot bath or shower and prepare to go to sleep.

You might feel tired, achy, or just generally exhausted. One reason is that nicotine sped up your metabolism and affected your sleeping patterns. Without nicotine, your body's rhythms are slowly starting to return to normal. If you feel tired, give in to that feeling. Go to sleep earlier than usual, because you need extra sleep and besides, while you're sleeping you're not smoking.

Don't forget to congratulate yourself when you've reached this point. You've made it! You've survived without cigarettes for one entire day, and each new day will be a little easier than the day before.

THE PERSONAL NUTRITION MANAGEMENT MENU PLANS

The Personal Nutrition Management Plan for weight loss is concerned not only with calories, but also with the *balance* of calories from carbohydrates, protein, fat, cholesterol, and sodium, as well as healthy amounts of fiber. There are five key guidelines to the menu plans that follow:

1. Limit dietary fat to between 20 to 30 percent of total calories, keep saturated fat below 10 percent, and emphasize monoun-saturated fats from olive oil, avocado, and nuts.
2. Eat minimally processed foods for a maximum feeling of fullness.
3. Eat at least five servings of fruit and/or vegetables per day.
4. Spread calories out so that you don't go more than four hours without eating. This applies to breakfast, lunch, dinner, and snacks.
5. Limit sweets, alcohol, and low-nutrient dense foods to 10 percent or less of total calories.

USING THE MENUS

Keep in mind that you are embarking on a long-term healthy eating plan—not a rigid diet.

These menus provide daily meal plans that can be eaten at home or ordered in a restaurant. You'll find three calorie levels: 1,500, 1,800, and 2,200. (To select your level, see page 70.) Those menu items marked with an asterisk (*) are included in the recipe collection in the back of the book. Week three is specifically designed for those who dine out frequently. Feel free to pick and choose and switch days around. This will ensure a balance of nutrients, particularly nutrients that are often low in new ex-smokers' diets. Repeat the menus until you make progress toward your goal and feel com-fortable with the new style of eating, or create your own menus using the book's recipes. How much weight you lose will depend on your metabolic rate and exercise level.

Go to Chapter 10 for general and specific information on ingredients. Then stock your cupboard and refrigerator according to the suggestions on pages 146–149. Soon you should be able to browse through the market and pick up whatever looks good, knowing that you'll be able to turn those items into nutritious, balanced meals.

Menu Plans / Week One

	BREAKFAST	LUNCH
SUNDAY 1,500 calories	Egg White Omelet with Green Onion and Parmesan,* 1 Orange Juice, 4 ounces Whole-Wheat Toast, 1 slice	Tex-Mex Bean and Cheese Burrito,* 1 Orange, 1
MONDAY 1,500 calories	Honey-Bran Blueberry Muffin,* 1	Leftover Best Grilled Swordfish,* 4 ounces, in Reduced-Fat Flour Tortilla with Salsa
TUESDAY 1,500 calories	Crunchy Granola,* ½ cup, or Equivalent 135-calorie Cereal	Lean Turkey Chili,* 1 cup Orange, 1 Fig Newton, 2, or Equivalent 100-Calorie Snack
WEDNESDAY 1,500 calories	Baked Oatmeal,* 1 serving Grapes, 1 cup	Barbecued Chicken Pizza,* 1 slice Basic Green Salad with Vinaigrette,* 1 serving Sliced Tomato Diet Soda or Water
THURSDAY 1,500 calories	Peanut Butter-Banana Toast,* 1 slice Grapefruit Juice, 4 ounces	Easy Ham and Cheese Quesadilla,* 1 serving Crunchy Oatmeal Chocolate Chip Cookies,* 2, or Equivalent 150-Calorie Snack
FRIDAY 1,500 calories	Ranch-Style Eggs with Tortillas,* 1 serving Sliced Tomato	Spinach and Zucchini Lasagna,* 1 serving Low-Fat Frozen Yogurt, 1 small cone
SATURDAY 1,500 calories	Buttermilk Pancakes,* 3 medium (5 inch) Maple Syrup, 4 tablespoons	Broiled Salmon with Garlic,* 4 ounces, with Salsa Lettuce Apple, 1, with Peanut Butter, 2 tablespoons

DINNER	SNACKS
Best Grilled Swordfish,* 4 ounces Tomato, Red Onion, and Avocado Salad,* 1 serving Cooked Rice, ½ cup, mixed with Salsa Crunchy Oatmeal Chocolate Chip Cookie,* 1	Low-Fat Frozen Yogurt, 1 small cone Banana, 1
Lean Turkey Chili,* 2 cups Cornbread (from Mix), ⅙ recipe Chewy Brownie,* 1, or Equivalent 100- Calorie Snack	Bagel Crisp, 1, with Cheese, 1 ounce Fresh Fruit in Season, 1 cup
Barbecued Chicken Pizza,* 2 slices Basic Green Salad with Vinaigrette,* 1 serving Easy Frozen Strawberry-Banana Pie,* 1 slice	Pretzels, 1½ ounces Chocolate Kisses, 2

Sweet and Sour Chicken Stir-Fry,*
    1 serving
Cooked Rice, ½ cup
Stir-Fried Snow Peas with Garlic and
    Ginger,* 1 serving
	Chewy Brownie,* 1, or Equivalent 100-
	    Calorie Snack
	Deli-Style Turkey Slices, 2 ounces, with
	Melon, 3 ounces

Spinach and Zucchini Lasagna,* 1 serving
Basic Green Salad with Vinaigrette,*
    1 serving
Chocolate Pudding,* ½ cup
	Refrigerator Buttermilk Bran Muffin,* 1, or
	    Equivalent 165-Calorie Snack
	Orange, 1

Broiled Salmon with Garlic,* 6 ounces Sautéed Zucchini with Garlic,* 1 serving Warm Potato Salad,* ¾ cup Chewy Brownies,* 1, or Equivalent 100- Calorie Snack	Apple, 1, with Cheddar Cheese, 1 ounce Light Ice Cream, ½ cup

Mustard-Glazed Pork Chop,* 1
Baked Potato, ½ small
Sautéed Green Beans with Walnuts and
    Lemon,* 1 cup
Chewy Brownie,* 1, or Equivalent 100-
    Calorie Snack
	Sliced Strawberries, 1 cup, with
	Brown Sugar, 1 teaspoon

Menu Plans / Week One

	BREAKFAST	LUNCH
SUNDAY 1,800 calories	Egg White Omelet with Green Onion and Parmesan,* 1 Grapefruit, ½ Whole-Wheat Toast, 2 slices Butter or Margarine, 2 teaspoons	Tex-Mex Bean and Cheese Burrito,* 1 Orange, 1 Crunchy Oatmeal Chocolate Chip Cookie,* 1
MONDAY 1,800 calories	Honey-Bran Blueberry Muffin,* 1 Banana or Papaya, 1, with Squeeze of Lemon and ½ cup Nonfat Yogurt	Leftover Best Grilled Swordfish,* 4 ounces, in Reduced-Fat Flour Tortilla with Salsa Crunchy Oatmeal Chocolate Chip Cookie,* 1, or Equivalent 75-Calorie Snack
TUESDAY 1,800 calories	Crunchy Granola,* ½ cup, or Equivalent 135-calorie Cereal Nonfat Milk, 8 ounces	Lean Turkey Chili,* 1 cup Orange, 1 Fig Newtons, 2, or Equivalent 100-Calorie Snack
WEDNESDAY 1,800 calories	Baked Oatmeal,* 1 serving Grapes, 1 cup	Barbecued Chicken Pizza,* 2 slices Basic Green Salad with Vinaigrette,* 1 serving Sliced Tomato Diet Soda or Water
THURSDAY 1,800 calories	Peanut Butter-Banana Toast,* 1 slice Grapefruit Juice, 8 ounces	Easy Ham and Cheese Quesadilla,* 1 serving Crunchy Oatmeal Chocolate Chip Cookie,* 1, or Equivalent 75-Calorie Snack
FRIDAY 1,800 calories	Ranch-Style Eggs with Tortillas,* 1 serving Sliced Tomato	Spinach and Zucchini Lasagna,* 1 serving Low-Fat Frozen Yogurt, 1 small cone
SATURDAY 1,800 calories	Buttermilk Pancakes,* 4 medium (5 inch) Maple Syrup, 2 tablespoons	Broiled Salmon with Garlic,* 4 ounces, in Reduced-Fat Flour Tortilla with Salsa Lettuce Apple, 1, with Peanut Butter, 2 tablespoons

DINNER	SNACKS
Best Grilled Swordfish,* 8 ounces Tomato, Red Onion, and Avocado Salad,* 1 serving Cooked Rice, ½ cup, mixed with Salsa Crunchy Oatmeal Chocolate Chip Cookies,* 2	Low-Fat Frozen Yogurt, 1 small cone Banana, 1 Crunchy Granola,* ½ cup
Lean Turkey Chili,* 2 cups Cornbread (from Mix), ⅙ recipe Chewy Brownie,* 1, or Equivalent 100- Calorie Snack	Bagel Crisp, 1, with Cheese, 1 ounce Fresh Fruit in Season, 1 cup
Barbecued Chicken Pizza,* 3 slices Basic Green Salad with Vinaigrette,* 1 serving Easy Frozen Strawberry-Banana Pie,* 1 slice	Pretzels, 1½ ounces Chocolate Kisses, 4

Sweet and Sour Chicken Stir-Fry,* 1 serving
Cooked Rice, 1 cup
Stir-Fried Snow Peas with Garlic and
   Ginger,* 1 serving
Melon Popsicle,* 1
	Chewy Brownie,* 1, or Equivalent 100-
	   Calorie Snack
	Deli-Style Turkey Slices, 2 ounces, with
	Melon, 3 ounces

Spinach and Zucchini Lasagna,*
   2 servings
Basic Green Salad with Vinaigrette,*
   1 serving
Chocolate Pudding,* ½ cup
	Refrigerator Buttermilk Bran Muffin,* 1, or
	   Equivalent 165-Calorie Snack
	Orange, 1

Broiled Salmon with Garlic,* 6 ounces Sautéed Zucchini with Garlic,* 1 serving Warm Potato Salad,* ¾ cup Chewy Brownies,* 1, or Equivalent 100- Calorie Snack	Apple, 1, with Cheddar Cheese, 1½ ounces Light Ice Cream, ½ cup

Mustard-Glazed Pork Chop,* 1
Baked Potato, 1 small
Sautéed Green Beans with Walnuts and
   Lemon,* 1 cup
Chewy Brownie,* 1, or Equivalent 100-
   Calorie Snack
	Crunchy Granola,* ½ cup, or Equivalent
	   135-Calorie Snack
	Sliced Strawberries, 1 cup, with
	Brown Sugar, 1 teaspoon

Menu Plans / Week One

	BREAKFAST	LUNCH
SUNDAY 2,200 calories	Egg White Omelet with Green Onion and Parmesan, * 1 Orange Juice, 8 ounces Whole-Wheat Toast, 2 slices Butter or Margarine, 2 teaspoons	Tex-Mex Bean and Cheese Burrito,* 1 Orange, 1
MONDAY 2,200 calories	Honey-Bran Blueberry Muffins,* 2 Banana or Papaya, 1, with Squeeze of Lemon and 1 cup Nonfat Yogurt	Leftover Best Grilled Swordfish,* 4 ounces, in Reduced-Fat Flour Tortillas, 2, with Salsa
TUESDAY 2,200 calories	Crunchy Granola,* 1½ cups, or Equivalent 300-Calorie Cereal Apple, 1	Lean Turkey Chili,* 1 cup Orange, 1 Fig Newtons, 3, or Equivalent 150-Calorie Snack
WEDNESDAY 2,200 calories	Baked Oatmeal,* 1 serving Grapes, 1 cup	Barbecued Chicken Pizza,* 3 slices Basic Green Salad with Vinaigrette,* 1 serving Sliced Tomato Diet Soda or Water
THURSDAY 2,200 calories	Peanut Butter-Banana Toast,* 1 slice Grapefruit Juice, 12 ounces	Easy Ham and Cheese Quesadillas,* 2 servings Crunchy Oatmeal Chocolate Chip Cookies,* 3, or Equivalent 225-Calorie Snack
FRIDAY 2,200 calories	Ranch-Style Eggs with Tortillas,* 1 serving Sliced Tomato Orange Juice, 8 ounces	Spinach and Zucchini Lasagna,* 1 serving Low-Fat Frozen Yogurt, 1 small cone
SATURDAY 2,200 calories	Buttermilk Pancakes,* 6 medium (5 inch) Maple Syrup, ¼ cup Nonfat Milk, 8 ounces	Broiled Salmon with Garlic,* 4 ounces, in Reduced-Fat Flour Tortilla with Salsa Lettuce Apple, 1, with Peanut Butter, 2 tablespoons

DINNER	SNACKS
Best Grilled Swordfish,* 8 ounces Tomato, Red Onion, and Avocado Salad,* 　　1 serving Cooked Rice, 1 cup, mixed with Salsa Crunchy Oatmeal Chocolate Chip Cookies,* 2	Low-Fat Frozen Yogurt, 1 small cone Banana, 1 Crunchy Granola,* 1 cup
Lean Turkey Chili,* 2 cups Cornbread (from Mix), ⅓ recipe Chewy Brownie,* 1, or Equivalent 100- 　　Calorie Snack	Bagel Crisps, 2, with Cheese, 1 ounce Fresh Fruit in Season, 1½ cups
Barbecued Chicken Pizza,* 3 slices Basic Green Salad with Vinaigrette,* 　　1 serving Easy Frozen Strawberry-Banana Pie,* 1 slice	Pretzels, 2 ounces Chocolate Kisses, 4
Sweet and Sour Chicken Stir-Fry,* 　　1½ servings Cooked Rice, 1 cup Stir-Fried Snow Peas with Garlic and 　　Ginger,* 1 serving Melon Popsicle,* 1	Chewy Brownie,* 1, or Equivalent 100- 　　Calorie Snack Deli-Style Turkey Slices, 2 ounces, with Melon, 3 ounces
Spinach and Zucchini Lasagna,* 　　2 servings Basic Green Salad with Vinaigrette,* 　　1 serving Chocolate Pudding,* ½ cup	Refrigerator Buttermilk Bran Muffin,* 1, or 　　Equivalent 165-Calorie Snack Orange, 1
Broiled Salmon with Garlic,* 6 ounces Sautéed Zucchini with Garlic,* 1 serving Warm Potato Salad,* 1 cup Chewy Brownies,* 2, or Equivalent 200- 　　Calorie Snack	Apple, 1, with Cheddar Cheese, 1½ ounces Light Ice Cream, ½ cup Mixed Nuts, ¼ cup
Mustard-Glazed Pork Chops,* 1 Baked Potato, 1 small Sautéed Green Beans with Walnuts and 　　Lemon,* 1 cup Chewy Brownies,* 2, or Equivalent 200- 　　Calorie Snack	Sliced Strawberries, 1 cup, with Brown Sugar, 1 teaspoon

Menu Plans / Week Two

	BREAKFAST	LUNCH
SUNDAY 1,500 calories	Refrigerator Buttermilk Bran Muffin,* 1, or Equivalent 165-Calorie Snack Nonfat Milk, 8 ounces Orange, 1	Easy Ham and Cheese Quesadilla,* 1 serving Apple, 1 Crunchy Oatmeal Chocolate Chip Cookie,* 1, or Equivalent 75-Calorie Snack
MONDAY 1,500 calories	Orange-Banana Breakfast Shake,* 1 Peanut Butter, 1 tablespoon	Corn Chowder,* 2 cups Nonfat Milk, 8 ounces Fig Newton, 1, or Equivalent 50-Calorie Snack
TUESDAY 1,500 calories	Sliced Strawberries, 1 cup Nonfat Yogurt, 1 cup Wheat Germ, 1 tablespoon	Leftover Cuban-Style Turkey in Tortillas,* 1 serving Shredded Cabbage Chewy Brownie,* 1, or Equivalent 100-Calorie Snack
WEDNESDAY 1,500 calories	Egg White Omelet with Green Onions and Parmesan,* 1 Orange Juice, 8 ounces	Chicken with Peas,* 1 serving Baked Potato, 1, with Nonfat Sour Cream, 1 tablespoon Tomato, ½ Easy Frozen Strawberry-Banana Pie,* 1 slice
THURSDAY 1,500 calories	Refrigerator Buttermilk Bran Muffin,* 1, or Equivalent 150-Calorie Muffin or Bread Grapefruit, 1, with Sugar, 1 teaspoon	Bagel with Cream Cheese and Salmon,* 1 serving Crunchy Oatmeal Chocolate Chip Cookie,* 1, or Equivalent 75-Calorie Snack
FRIDAY 1,500 calories	Cooked Oatmeal, ¾ cup Maple Syrup or Brown Sugar, 1 tablespoon Grapefruit Juice, 8 ounces	Old-Fashioned Beef Stew,* 2 cups Apple, 1
SATURDAY 1,500 calories	French Toast,* 1 slice Banana, ½	Sandwich: Multigrain Bread, 2 slices, with Tomato, ½; Avocado, ¼; Lettuce; Part-Skim Mozzarella, 1 ounce; and Low-Fat Mayonnaise, 1 tablespoon Chocolate Birthday Cake,* 1 slice, or Equivalent 200-Calorie Snack

DINNER	SNACKS
Corn Chowder,* 2 cups Whole-Wheat Toast, 1 slice Part-Skim Mozzarella, 2 ounces Crunchy Oatmeal Chocolate Chip Cookies,* 2, or Equivalent 150-Calorie Snack	Grapes, 1 cup
Cuban-Style Turkey in Tortillas,* 1 serving Cooked Rice, ½ cup Salsa Chewy Brownie,* 1, or Equivalent 100- Calorie Snack	Apple, 1 Nonfat Fruited Yogurt, 1 cup
Chicken with Peas,* 1 serving Cooked Rice, 1 cup Low-Fat Frozen Yogurt, ½ cup Peach, 1	Crunchy Granola,* ½ cup, or Equivalent 135-Calorie Snack
Grilled Fish with Tomato Salsa,* 6 ounces Reduced-Fat Flour Tortilla, 1 Black Beans, ¾ cup	Easy Frozen Strawberry-Banana Pie,* 1 slice
Old-Fashioned Beef Stew,* 1 serving Chocolate Pudding,* ½ cup	Deli-Style Turkey Slices, 2 ounces, with Melon, 3 ounces Air-Popped Popcorn, 3 cups
Barbecued Chicken Chopped Salad,* 1 serving	Dried Apricots, 10 Mixed Nuts, ¼ cup
Chicken Parmesan with Pasta,* 1 serving Extra Cooked Pasta, ½ cup Wilted Spinach Salad,* 1 serving Parmesan Cheese, 2 tablespoons	Frozen Banana "Ice Cream,"* 1 serving

Menu Plans / Week Two

	BREAKFAST	LUNCH
SUNDAY 1,800 calories	Refrigerator Buttermilk Bran Muffins,* 2, or Equivalent 165-Calorie Each Muffin Nonfat Milk, 8 ounces Orange, 1	Easy Ham and Cheese Quesadilla,* 1 serving Apple, 1 Crunchy Oatmeal Chocolate Chip Cookie,* 1, or Equivalent 75-Calorie Snack
MONDAY 1,800 calories	Orange-Banana Breakfast Shake,* 1 Whole-Wheat Toast, 1 slice Peanut Butter, 1 tablespoon	Corn Chowder,* 2 cups Nonfat Milk, 8 ounces Fig Newtons, 2, or Equivalent 100-Calorie Snack
TUESDAY 1,800 calories	Banana, 1 Sliced Strawberries, 1 cup Nonfat Yogurt, 1 cup Wheat Germ, 1 tablespoon	Leftover Cuban-Style Turkey in Tortillas,* 1 serving Shredded Cabbage Chewy Brownie,* 1, or Equivalent 100-Calorie Snack
WEDNESDAY 1,800 calories	Egg White Omelet with Green Onions and Parmesan,* 1 Whole-Grain Toast, 1 slice Orange Juice, 8 ounces	Chicken with Peas,* 1 serving Baked Potato, 1, with Nonfat Sour Cream, 1 tablespoon Tomato, ½ Easy Frozen Strawberry-Banana Pie,* 1 slice
THURSDAY 1,800 calories	Refrigerator Buttermilk Bran Muffins,* 2, or Equivalent 150-Calorie Each Muffin or Bread Grapefruit, ½, with Sugar, 1 teaspoon	Bagel with Cream Cheese and Salmon,* 1 serving Banana, 1 Crunchy Oatmeal Chocolate Chip Cookie,* 1, or Equivalent 75-Calorie Snack
FRIDAY 1,800 calories	Cooked Oatmeal, 1 cup Maple Syrup or Brown Sugar, 1 tablespoon Banana, 1	Old-Fashioned Beef Stew,* 2 cups Apple, 1
SATURDAY 1,800 calories	French Toast,* 1 slice Banana, 1	Sandwich: Multigrain Bread, 2 slices; with Tomato, ½; Avocado, ¼; Lettuce; Part-Skim Mozzarella, 1 ounce; and Low-Fat Mayonnaise, 1 tablespoon Chocolate Birthday Cake,* 1 slice, or Equivalent 200-Calorie Snack

DINNER	SNACKS
Corn Chowder,* 2 cups Whole-Wheat Toast, 1 slice Part-Skim Mozzarella, 2 ounces Crunchy Oatmeal Chocolate Chip Cookies,* 2, or Equivalent 150-Calorie Snack	Grapes, 1 cup Peanuts, ¼ cup

Cuban-Style Turkey in Tortillas,* 1 serving
Cooked Rice, ½ cup
Salsa
Chewy Brownie,* 1, or Equivalent 100-
    Calorie Snack
	Refrigerator Buttermilk Bran Muffin,* 1, or
	    Equivalent 165-Calorie Snack
	Apple, 1
	Nonfat Fruited Yogurt, 1 cup

Chicken with Peas,* 1 serving Cooked Rice, 1 cup Low-Fat Frozen Yogurt, 1 cup Peach, 1	Pretzels, 1½ ounces Crunchy Granola,* ½ cup, or Equivalent 135-Calorie Snack
Grilled Fish with Tomato Salsa,* 6 ounces Reduced-Fat Flour Tortillas, 2 Black Beans, 1 cup	Easy Frozen Strawberry-Banana Pie,* 1 slice Bagel Crisp, 1, with Cheese, 1 ounce
Old-Fashioned Beef Stew,* 2 cups Chocolate Pudding,* ½ cup	Deli-Style Turkey Slices, 2 ounces, with Melon, 3 ounces Air-Popped Popcorn, 3 cups

Barbecued Chicken Chopped Salad,*
    1 serving
Baked Corn Tortillas, 2, or Equivalent 170-
    Calorie Baked Tortilla Chips
Chocolate Birthday Cake,* 1 slice, or
    Equivalent 200-Calorie Snack
	Dried Apricots, 10
	Mixed Nuts, ¼ cup

Chicken Parmesan with Pasta,* 1 serving Extra Cooked Pasta, 1 cup Wilted Spinach Salad,* 1 serving Parmesan Cheese, 2 tablespoons	Frozen Banana "Ice Cream,"* 1 serving

Menu Plans / Week Two

	BREAKFAST	LUNCH
SUNDAY 2,200 calories	Refrigerator Buttermilk Bran Muffins,* 2, or Equivalent 165-Calorie Each Muffin Nonfat Milk, 8 ounces Orange, 1	Easy Ham and Cheese Quesadilla,* 1 serving Apple, 1 Crunchy Oatmeal Chocolate Chip Cookie,* 1, or Equivalent 75-Calorie Snack
MONDAY 2,200 calories	Orange-Banana Breakfast Shake,* 1 Whole-Wheat Toast, 2 slices Peanut Butter, 1 tablespoon	Corn Chowder,* 4 cups Nonfat Milk, 8 ounces Fig Newtons, 3, or Equivalent 150-Calorie Snack
TUESDAY 2,200 calories	Banana, 1 Sliced Strawberries, 1 cup Nonfat Yogurt, 1 cup Wheat Germ, 1 tablespoon	Leftover Cuban-Style Turkey in Tortillas,* 2 servings Shredded Cabbage Chewy Brownie,* 1, or Equivalent 100-Calorie Snack
WEDNESDAY 2,200 calories	Egg White Omelet with Green Onion and Parmesan,* 2 servings Whole-Grain Toast, 2 slices Orange Juice, 8 ounces	Chicken with Peas,* 1 serving Baked Potato, 1, with Nonfat Sour Cream, 1 tablespoon Tomato, 1 Easy Frozen Strawberry-Banana Pie,* 1 slice
THURSDAY 2,200 calories	Refrigerator Buttermilk Bran Muffins,* 2, or Equivalent 150-Calorie Each Muffin or Bread Grapefruit, 1, with Sugar, 1 teaspoon	Bagel with Cream Cheese and Salmon,* 1 serving Banana, 1 Crunchy Oatmeal Chocolate Chip Cookies,* 2, or Equivalent 150-Calorie Snack
FRIDAY 2,200 calories	Cooked Oatmeal, 1½ cups Maple Syrup or Brown Sugar, 2 tablespoons Banana, 1	Old-Fashioned Beef Stew,* 2 cups Apple, 1
SATURDAY 2,200 calories	French Toast,* 3 slices Banana, 1	Sandwich: Multigrain Bread, 2 slices, with Tomato, ½; Avocado, ¼; Lettuce; Part-Skim Mozzarella, 1 ounce; and Low-Fat Mayonnaise, 1 tablespoon Chocolate Birthday Cake,* 1 slice, or Equivalent 200-Calorie Snack

DINNER	SNACKS
Corn Chowder,* 4 cups Whole-Wheat Toast, 2 slices Part-Skim Mozzarella, 2 ounces Crunchy Oatmeal Chocolate Chip Cookies,* 2, or Equivalent 150-Calorie Snack	Grapes, 2 cups Peanuts, ¼ cup

Cuban-Style Turkey in Tortillas,* 1 serving
Cooked Rice, 1 cup
Salsa
Chewy Brownie,* 1, or Equivalent 100-
  Calorie Snack
	Refrigerator Buttermilk Bran Muffin,* 1, or
	  Equivalent 165-Calorie Snack
	Apple, 1
	Nonfat Fruited Yogurt, 1 cup

Chicken with Peas,* 1 serving Cooked Rice, 1 cup Low-Fat Frozen Yogurt, 1½ cups Peach, 1	Pretzels, 1½ ounces Crunchy Granola,* ½ cup, or Equivalent 135-Calorie Snack
Grilled Fish with Tomato Salsa,* 6 ounces Reduced-Fat Flour Tortillas, 2 Black Beans, 1 cup	Easy Frozen Strawberry-Banana Pie,* 1 slice Bagel Crisp, 1, with Cheese, 1 ounce Apple, 1
Old-Fashioned Beef Stew,* 3 cups Chocolate Pudding,* ½ cup	Deli-Style Turkey Slices, 4 ounces, with Melon, 4 ounces Air-Popped Popcorn, 3 cups

Barbecued Chicken Chopped Salad,*
  1½ servings
Baked Corn Tortillas, 2, or Equivalent 170-
  Calorie Baked Tortilla Chips
Chocolate Birthday Cake,* 1 slice, or
  Equivalent 200-Calorie Snack
	Dried Apricots, 10
	Mixed Nuts, ¼ cup

Chicken Parmesan with Pasta,* 1½ servings Extra Cooked Pasta, 1 cup Wilted Spinach Salad,* 1 serving Parmesan Cheese, 2 tablespoons	Frozen Banana "Ice Cream,"* 1 serving

Menu Plans / Week One–Eating Out

	BREAKFAST	LUNCH

SUNDAY
1,500 calories
	Bagel, ½ small
	Cream Cheese, 1 tablespoon
	Smoked Salmon, 2 ounces
	Orange Juice, 8 ounces, or
	  1 cup Fresh Fruit
		Turkey Deli Sandwich with mustard,
		  lettuce, and tomato, 1
		Chicken Noodle Soup, 1 cup
		Non-Calorie Beverage

MONDAY 1,500 calories	Nutrigrain Bar, 1 Nonfat Milk, 8 ounces	Chicken Caesar Salad (with Croutons), 1 serving Carrot Juice, 8 ounces

TUESDAY
1,500 calories
	Jamba Juice Fruit Smoothie
	  (300 calories or less), 1
		Turkey Deli Sandwich with Swiss
		  Cheese, Mustard, and Tomato on
		  Whole-Wheat Bread, 1
		Green Salad with Low-Calorie
		  Dressing

WEDNESDAY
1,500 calories
	Bran Flakes or Shredded Wheat,
	  1 cup
	Banana, ½
	Low-Fat Milk, 8 ounces
	Orange Juice, 8 ounces, or
	  1 cup Fresh Fruit
		Ham Sandwich on Rye Bread with
		  Mustard, Lettuce, and Tomato, 1
		Tomato Juice, 8 ounces

THURSDAY
1,500 calories
	Starbucks Power Frappuccino
	  (coffee flavored, 12 ounces), 1
		McDonald's Grilled Chicken Deluxe
		  (no mayonnaise), 1
		Garden Salad with Low-Calorie
		  Dressing
		Diet Soda
		Low-Fat Yogurt Cone, 1

FRIDAY
1,500 calories
	Oatmeal, 1 cup
	Banana, 1
	Raisins, ¼ cup
	Nonfat Milk, 8 ounces
	Grapefruit Juice, 8 ounces, or
	  1 cup Fresh Fruit
		Chinese Chicken Salad (without
		  fried crisps or wontons),
		  1 serving
		Non-Calorie Beverage

SATURDAY
1,500 calories
	Poached Egg, 1
	Whole-Wheat Toast, 1 slice
	Orange Juice, 8 ounces, or
	  1 cup Fresh Fruit
		Carl's Junior Roast Chicken
		  Sandwich, 1
		Diet Beverage
		Frozen Yogurt with Fresh Fruit
		  Topping, 1

DINNER	SNACKS
Angel Hair Pasta, 1 cup, with Tomato Sauce, ½ cup Green Salad with Grated Carrot and Vinaigrette Steamed Asparagus, 6 spears Fruit Sorbet, ½ cup	Low-Fat Yogurt Cone, 1 Fig Newtons, 2
Chicken Soft Taco or Chicken Burrito, 1 Rice, ½ cup Beans, ½ cup Water or Non-Calorie Beverage	Fig Newtons, 2 Mixed Nuts, ¼ cup Dried Apricots, 5
Shrimp with Snow Peas, 1 cup Rice, ⅓ cup Fortune Cookie, 1	Carrots and Celery with Fat-Free Ranch Dip Grapes or Cut Fresh Fruit, 1 cup Mixed Nuts, ¼ cup
Roasted Chicken (light meat, no skin), 4 ounces Starch Side (Roasted Potatoes, Rice), ½ cup Vegetable Side (Green Beans, Spinach, Carrots), ¾ cup	Light Ice Cream, ½ cup Fresh Berries, ½ cup Grapes, 1 cup
Pizza with Sliced Tomato and Garlic, Easy on Cheese, 1 slice Green Salad with Vinaigrette	Apple, 1, with Peanut Butter, 2 tablespoons Orange Juice, 8 ounces Chocolate Kisses, 4
Mixed Sushi and Sushi Rolls, 6 pieces Miso Soup, 1 cup Cucumber Salad	Carrots, 2 Orange, 1 Biscotti, 1
Teriyaki Chicken (no skin), 4 ounces Rice Pilaf, 1 cup Grilled Pineapple, ½ cup Vegetable Side, 1 cup	Banana, 1 Low-Fat Frozen Yogurt, ½ cup Fresh Pineapple Chunks, ½ cup Nonfat Milk, 8 ounces

Menu Plans / Week One–Eating Out

	BREAKFAST	LUNCH
SUNDAY 1,800 calories	Bagel, 1 small, or ½ large Cream Cheese, 1 tablespoon Smoked Salmon, 2 ounces Orange Juice, 8 ounces, or 1 cup Fresh Fruit	Turkey Deli Sandwich with Mustard, Lettuce, and Tomato, 1 Chicken Noodle Soup, 1 cup Non-Calorie Beverage
MONDAY 1,800 calories	Nutrigrain Bars, 2 Nonfat Milk, 8 ounces	Chicken Caesar Salad (with Croutons), 1 serving Carrot Juice, 8 ounces
TUESDAY 1,800 calories	Jamba Juice Fruit Smoothie (400 calories or less), 1	Turkey Deli Sandwich with Swiss Cheese, Mustard, and Tomato on Whole-Wheat Bread, 1 Green Salad with Low-Calorie Dressing
WEDNESDAY 1,800 calories	Bran Flakes or Shredded Wheat, 1 cup Banana, ½ Low-Fat Milk, 8 ounces Orange Juice, 8 ounces, or 1 cup Fresh Fruit	Ham Sandwich on Rye Bread with Mustard, Lettuce, and Tomato, 1 Tomato Juice, 8 ounces
THURSDAY 1,800 calories	Starbucks Power Frappuccino (coffee flavored, 16 ounces), 1	McDonald's Grilled Chicken Deluxe (no mayonnaise), 1 Garden Salad with Low-Calorie Dressing Diet Soda Low-Fat Yogurt Cone, 1
FRIDAY 1,800 calories	Oatmeal, 1 cup Banana, 1 Raisins, ¼ cup Nonfat Milk, 8 ounces Grapefruit Juice, 8 ounces, or 1 cup Fresh Fruit	Chinese Chicken Salad (without fried crisps or wontons), 1 serving Non-Calorie Beverage
SATURDAY 1,800 calories	Poached Eggs, 2 Whole-Wheat Toast, 2 slices Orange Juice, 8 ounces, or 1 cup Fresh Fruit	Carl's Junior Roast Chicken Sandwich, 1 Diet Beverage Frozen Yogurt with Fresh Fruit Topping, 1

DINNER	SNACKS
Angel Hair Pasta, 1 cup, with Tomato Sauce, ½ cup Green Salad with Grated Carrot and Vinaigrette Steamed Asparagus, 6 spears Fruit Sorbet, ½ cup	Banana, 1 Low-Fat Yogurt Cone, 1 Fig Newtons, 2
Chicken Soft Taco or Chicken Burrito, 1 Rice, ½ cup Beans, ½ cup Water or Non-Calorie Beverage	Fig Newtons, 2 Mixed Nuts, ¼ cup Dried Apricots, 10
Shrimp with Snow Peas, 1½ cups Rice, ⅓ cup Fortune Cookies, 2	Carrots and Celery with Fat-Free Ranch Dip Grapes or Cut Fresh Fruit, 1 cup Mixed Nuts, ¼ cup
Roasted Chicken (light meat, no skin), 6 ounces Starch Side (Roasted Potatoes, Rice), 1 cup Vegetable Side (Green Beans, Spinach, Carrots), 1 cup	Light Ice Cream, ½ cup Fresh Berries, 1 cup Grapes, 1 cup Mixed Nuts, ¼ cup
Pizza with Sliced Tomato and Garlic, Easy on Cheese, 2 slices Green Salad with Vinaigrette	Apple, 1, with Peanut Butter, 2 tablespoons Orange Juice, 8 ounces Chocolate Kisses, 4
Mixed Sushi and Sushi Rolls, 10 pieces Miso Soup, 1 cup Cucumber Salad	Carrots, 2 Orange, 1 Biscotti, 2
Teriyaki Chicken (no skin), 1½ cups Rice Pilaf, 1 cup Grilled Pineapple, ½ cup Vegetable Side, 1 cup	Fresh Fruit, 1 piece Animal Crackers, 1 box Nonfat Milk, 8 ounces

Menu Plans / Week One–Eating Out

	BREAKFAST	LUNCH

SUNDAY
2,200 calories
	Bagel, 1 small, or ½ large
	Cream Cheese, 1 tablespoon
	Smoked Salmon, 2 ounces
	Orange Juice, 8 ounces, or
	  1 cup Fresh Fruit
		Turkey Deli Sandwich with mustard,
		  lettuce, and tomato, 1
		Chicken Noodle Soup, 1 cup
		Non-Calorie Beverage

MONDAY 2,200 calories	Nutrigrain Bars, 2 Nonfat Milk, 8 ounces	Chicken Caesar Salad (with Croutons), 1½ servings Carrot Juice, 12 ounces

TUESDAY
2,200 calories
	Jamba Juice Fruit Smoothie
	(400 calories or less), 1
		Turkey Deli Sandwich with Swiss
		  Cheese, Mustard, and Tomato on
		  Whole-Wheat Bread, 1
		Green Salad with Low-Calorie
		  Dressing

WEDNESDAY
2,200 calories
	Bran Flakes or Shredded Wheat,
	  1½ cups
	Banana, 1
	Low-Fat Milk, 8 ounces
	Orange Juice, 8 ounces, or
	  1 cup Fresh Fruit
		Ham Sandwich on Rye Bread with
		  Mustard, Lettuce, and Tomato, 1
		Tomato Juice, 8 ounces

THURSDAY
2,200 calories
	Starbuck's Power Frappuccino
	(coffee flavored, 20 ounces), 1
		McDonald's Grilled Chicken Deluxe
		  (no mayonnaise), 1
		Garden Salad with Low-Calorie
		  Dressing
		Diet Soda
		Low-Fat Yogurt Cone, 1

FRIDAY
2,200 calories
	Oatmeal, 1½ cups
	Banana, 1
	Raisins, ¼ cup
	Nonfat Milk, 8 ounces
	Grapefruit Juice, 4 ounces
		Chinese Chicken Salad (without
		  fried crisps or wontons),
		  1½ servings
		Non-Calorie Beverage

SATURDAY
2,200 calories
	Poached Eggs, 2
	Whole-Wheat Toast, 2 slices
	Orange Juice, 8 ounces, or
	  1 cup Fresh Fruit
		Carl's Junior Roast Chicken
		  Sandwich, 1
		Diet Beverage
		Low-Fat Frozen Yogurt with Fresh
		  Fruit Topping, 1

DINNER	SNACKS
Angel Hair Pasta, 2 cups, with Tomato Sauce, 1 cup Green Salad with Grated Carrot and Vinaigrette Steamed Asparagus, 6 spears Fruit Sorbet, ½ cup	Banana, 1 Low-Fat Yogurt Cone, 1 Fig Newtons, 2
Chicken Soft Tacos, or Chicken Burritos, 2 Rice, ¾ cup Beans, ½ cup Water or Non-Calorie Beverage	Fig Newtons, 4 Mixed Nuts, ¼ cup Dried Apricots, 10
Shrimp with Snow Peas, 2 cups Rice, 1 cup Fortune Cookies, 2	Carrots and Celery with Fat-Free Ranch Dip Grapes or Cut Fresh Fruit, 1 cup Mixed Nuts, ¼ cup
Roasted Chicken (light meat, no skin), 12 ounces Starch Side (Roasted Potatoes, Rice), 1 cup Vegetable Side (Green Beans, Spinach, Carrots), 1½ cups	Light Ice Cream, ½ cup Fresh Berries, 1 cup Grapes, 2 cups Mixed Nuts, ¼ cup
Pizza with Sliced Tomato and Garlic, Easy on Cheese, 3 slices Green Salad with Vinaigrette	Apple, 1, with Peanut Butter, 2 tablespoons Orange Juice, 8 ounces Chocolate Kisses, 10 Banana, 1
Mixed Sushi and Sushi Rolls, 12 pieces Miso Soup, 1 cup Cucumber Salad	Carrots, 2 Orange, 1 Bagel, ½ with Cream Cheese, 1 tablespoon Biscotti, 2
Teriyaki Chicken (no skin), 1½ cups Rice Pilaf, 1½ cups Grilled Pineapple, 1 cup Vegetable Side, 1 cup	Cut Fresh Fruit, 1½ cups Nonfat Milk, 8 ounces

CHAPTER 6
Motivation:
Change Your
Thoughts, Change
Your Behavior

Addiction is like a triangle, and overcoming the chemical addiction is just one of the three sides. The other two sides—changing your behavior and tackling the psychological reasons for dependence—must also be dealt with if you are to quit smoking permanently. A parallel set of steps can provide you with the motivation you need to stop smoking—and help change your eating behavior as well.

According to Dr. Anthony Reading, associate clinical professor of psychiatry at the University of California, Los Angeles, one of the big myths of smoking cessation is that willpower will see you through. "Willpower doesn't carry you for twenty-four hours. You need motivation, which is the perception that one is capable of achieving a target and possesses the skills to move to that target."

Motivation is not some mysterious thing that sometimes happens and sometimes doesn't, although it often feels that way. Think of it like a computer program. Some psychologists suggest that a human being is essentially an information processing "machine" and thought patterns are just the programs being processed. To get the right outcome—the motivation to stay off tobacco—you need to be programmed correctly.

Sometimes, by design or accident, we run the right program and finish what we set out to accomplish. In those cases, we refer to ourselves as having been sufficiently motivated. When we don't finish a project, or perhaps never even start, we say that we lacked motivation. Another way of looking at it, however, is to consider that we didn't "enter in" the right thoughts or run the right program, or perhaps we never learned the program.

How we think can affect the way we behave. If we expect to fail, chances are we will fail, whether our goal is quitting smoking or eating more health-fully. Negative thoughts increase stress and anxiety, and put a damper on our self-esteem, which is a sure way to go back to the behaviors that got us in trouble in the first place. Here's some practical help. Whenever you catch a negative thought floating through your mind, replace it with a positive yet realistic statement. The idea is not to deny what you're feeling, but to see your situation from another perspective.

One way to subtly induce failure is to create unrealistic expectations. If you set the bar too high, you're bound to fail. It might take only a day or two before you abandon your goals and binge on a bag of cookies or reach for a pack of cigarettes. In both cases, negative behavior reaffirms negative thought patterns, which are generated by your nicotine addiction. Setting realistic goals for yourself is a good way to avoid this negative feedback loop. Especially during this transitional period in your life, make sure that you are your own best friend rather than a taskmaster.

Here are some examples of ways to overcome negative, punishing thought patterns and turn unrealistic expectations into positive, achievable goals.

Old Script	New Script
1. From now on, I'm going to avoid all sweets and desserts, especially chocolate chip cookies.	Although total abstinence works with cigarettes, food is different. I need to eat, and my body naturally craves sweets. (For more on cravings, see page 38.) I can learn to eat chocolate chip cookies in moderation, but until I do, I'll avoid them. Eventually I will learn to control my cravings instead of being controlled by them.

Old Script	New Script
2. Never again will I overeat.	It's time to be more flexible with myself; everyone overeats occasionally. If I do, it doesn't mean that I've sabotaged all my efforts to lose weight or avoid gaining. My objective is to make wise food choices *most* of the time and to avoid overeating whenever possible. (See Chapter 8 for more on overeating.) In this way, I'll avoid the yo-yo effect of going to extremes.
3. I'm not going to gain a single pound when I quit smoking.	Although this sounds like a good goal, it's too abstract. To avoid weight gain I need to be specific and focus on what I must *do,* like making sensible food choices, eating moderate portions, and exercising regularly. I might even need to allow myself to gain a few pounds without becoming overwhelmed, and then focus on weight loss.

Old Script

4. I'm going to exercise every day.

5. I've been trying to lose weight all my life and I guess I'm just destined to be fat.

6. I'm gaining weight in spite of all my efforts; I must be doing something wrong.

New Script

This also sounds great, but it might not be realistic. I'm going to try to exercise at least every other day, or not miss exercising more than two days in a row. If I get more than that, all the better. I'll try to achieve a regular pattern of exercise that suits my schedule and lifestyle. Each session will be at least 15 to 20 minutes in order to get all the benefits of aerobic exercise.

I must beware of predicting a result—it may become a self-fulfilling prophecy. Perhaps the restrictive diets I've tried in the past set me up to fail. This isn't just about avoiding weight gain, it's about a new approach to life that will make me healthier. I need to take it one day at a time, and I'll reach my goals.

I need to take a closer look at my choices and be honest with myself. Am I eating more calories than I need? Am I exercising enough? Am I finding the right balance between food intake, food choices, and decreased calories, while still satisfying my appetite? I can counteract the effects of eating a little bit more one day by exercising a little bit more another day. If I make the right choices, I won't automatically gain weight.

Old Script	New Script
7. Poor me! First I have to give up cigarettes; now I have to give up all my favorite foods.	I must stop feeling sorry for myself and stay focused on my goals. I've already begun to appreciate the health benefits of not smoking. Soon I'll train myself to be satisfied with smaller portions of sweets and high-calorie foods while learning to enjoy the flavors of fruits, vegetables, whole grains, lean meats, and low-fat dairy products.
8. With my demanding job and schedule (not to mention my mother or my spouse or my kids), it's impossible to eat right.	My job is intense, but it's no excuse to overeat or relapse back to smoking. I need to be more creative about finding a restaurant nearby that offers better choices, or keep healthy foods at the office so I avoid getting too hungry, which is a sure trigger to overeat and to smoke. As for my family, I need to be assertive in letting them know how they can support me. Quitting smoking is good for me, and that's good for all of us.
9. Being on a diet is boring and all my friends won't want to be around me. I'm no fun anymore.	I can enjoy a dinner out without overeating. In fact, if I don't say anything, no one is likely to know, or even care, that I'm choosing different foods than usual. I can simply say, "This food is delicious," or "I'm so full, I couldn't eat another bite." My dietary choices don't need to be conversation fodder. Talking about it is not important—*doing* is what counts.

Old Script	New Script
10. What if I do gain weight when I quit smoking? I would hate myself and start smoking again.	I may have ups and downs with my weight, but I need to learn to deal with these small fluctuations. If I carefully consider what I'm eating, I can see when I'm taking too big a portion at dinner, or getting too many calories from snacks, and cut back. The numbers on the scale are something I can learn from, not evidence that I can't cope with.

Remember that part of what keeps fit people fit is their ability to pick themselves up and get going again after a period of too little exercise and too much food. *Starting smoking again is not the answer.* You would have to gain over 100 pounds to equal the health risks of smoking just one pack per day!

11. What if this program doesn't work?	Whether or not I gain weight does not really depend on this program, it depends on me. If I make wise food choices most of the time and get enough exercise, I will manage my weight.
12. I don't have the willpower to make changes.	Willpower is elusive and cannot be relied upon. Instead, I need to learn what to do, decide on a plan, and find a way to make it fit into my life. I'll set realistic goals and take small steps to get there.

Old Script	New Script
13. I'm craving a sweet and I just can't resist.	It's normal to crave sweets, particularly when I'm going through nicotine withdrawal. But it only takes a small amount of the desired food to satisfy true biological cravings. (See page 38.) To make sure it's biological and not emotional, I'll delay eating for 10 minutes, make a phone call or take a bath, and then see if I still need to eat. If I do, I'll have a small amount to satisfy my craving, without going overboard.
14. I'm so hungry, I've got to eat.	It's okay to eat when I'm hungry. Hunger is a natural response when the body needs energy. If I eat when I'm hungry and stop when I'm full I won't have a problem. I need to be careful not to get overly hungry though, because that can make me lose control and overeat.
15. It tastes so good, I'd like some more.	Part of my new behavior is to stop eating when I've had enough. How much is enough? This literally depends on the volume of food in my stomach. I'll check portion sizes and remember that second helpings of high-calorie foods quickly become "excess baggage." Since it takes about 20 minutes for my brain to get the message

Old Script

New Script

that my stomach's full, I'll slow
down while eating and pace
myself. I know it's hard to resist
things that taste so good, but I
don't have to give in—my
willpower can be stronger than
my cravings. I'll have a cup of
decaffeinated coffee or some water
instead and put the food out of my
sight as soon as possible.

16. Quitting smoking is so stressful, I can't manage my weight
on top of it.

I can use food to help me cope as
long as I balance my food choices
and avoid overeating. Food is a
treat for me, but I must find other
non-food treats.

I will work on incorporating
stress-reducing activities into my
life, such as deep-breathing exercises, taking long walks, enjoying a
relaxing hot bath, or going to a
movie. I will talk over my feelings
with a friend or a "stop smoking"
buddy. I'll realize that lighting up
doesn't really remove the ultimate
cause of my stress, it just buries it
underneath a layer of chemicals in
the brain. Nothing changes by giving in to nicotine.

Old Script	New Script
17. When I'm at a restaurant or someone's house and I'm served a plate of food, I must clean my plate.	I can be more liberal with *what* I eat if I can pay better attention to *how much* I eat. I need to remember that I can overeat with healthy foods, too. If I'm at a restaurant, I'll ask the server to wrap up what's left before I find myself finishing every-thing off. Or I can simply ask the server to take my plate away. If I'm at someone's house, I'll explain that the meal was absolutely delicious, but I'm already full.
18. I blew it today; I may as well give up.	Just because I ate too much today doesn't mean I should abandon all my efforts. I'm only human and everyone has eating indiscretions now and then; it's how I react to them that will make the difference. I'll get back on track at the next meal.
19. I'm too tired to cook.	I might not feel like cooking every night, but I have a back-up plan: healthful frozen dinners or take-out food.

Old Script	New Script
20. I'm craving it, so my body must need it.	The body does not become addicted to food the way it does to nicotine, but eating certain sugary foods can elevate chemicals in the brain and make us feel less stressed. The good news is that it takes only a small amount of those foods to satisfy the craving. I can go ahead and honor my craving if I remember to *eat a small portion.*

These are just a few of the ways to turn negative thoughts and unrealistic expectations on their head. Replacing self-defeating prophecies with positive messages can be just as important as exercise and working with your diet. Once you expect to succeed, success is more likely to be yours. Stop asking WHY you aren't motivated and start asking HOW you can motivate yourself.

CHAPTER 7
Exercise Is Key

Gaining weight after you stop smoking appears to be due to a combination of factors, most notably an increased intake of calories and a slowing of the body's metabolic rate. The fact that your metabolism decreases when you stop smoking suggests that even people who don't increase their food intake may still gain some weight in the process. Happily, there's a simple remedy for this potential problem—exercise.

Exercise is an essential piece of the new ex-smoker's weight-control equation. It's the one sure way to offset any increase in calories that results from your slowed metabolism. If you were burning an extra 200 calories per day by smoking cigarettes, for example, simply increase your daily exercise level by 200 calories to compensate. Exercise is also an excellent way to cope with feelings of irritability and anger as well as the daily buildup of stress that many smokers experience right after quitting.

Here's another great reason to exercise: If you lose weight from calorie restriction alone, it's likely that 65 percent of that loss will involve muscle. That means 10 pounds of overall weight loss nets only 3½ pounds of fat loss; the rest comes from vital muscle stores. This can be particularly bad news for new ex-smokers because less muscle mass means less metabolic activity, which will exacerbate the already dropping metabolic rate they experience from nicotine withdrawal.

Not all researchers agree that eliminating nicotine means you'll require 200 fewer calories per day. They do agree, however, that you'll have more energy available as soon as you stop smoking because poisonous carbon monoxide won't be entering your lungs and bloodstream. Don't worry if you find yourself coughing more during the first few weeks. That's just the cilia (tiny hairlike fingers that line the airways) in your lungs beginning to work again. Your entire body is waking up, replenishing itself, and starting to live again. (Having a relapse and smoking even one cigarette will interrupt the process and filling your lungs with carbon monoxide.)

Common sense suggests that it's easier to burn calories when you're not smoking than when you are. As your body rids itself of carbon monoxide, your red blood cells (hemoglobin) will become saturated with oxygen so that you don't get winded as quickly as you used to, and you have significantly more energy than you ever did when you were smoking. Go out and take a walk—you'll find that everything just seems to work better. Your lungs will feel stronger, your breathing will return to a healthier level of activity—this rejuvenating process begins the moment you quit cigarettes for good, and exercise only makes it better.

EXERCISE GETS RESULTS

When you quit smoking, the initial exercise goal is to offset the presumed 200 calories that are added to your system each day as a result of your slowed metabolic rate. Here's a good rule to remember: Walking one mile burns up about 100 calories for a 150-pound person. It takes around 20 minutes to walk a mile, so walking for about 40 minutes to walk two miles will burn 200 calories. If you weigh more or less, divide your weight by 150, then multiply that number by 100 to determine how many calories you'll burn. For example, a person weighing 300 pounds uses 200 calories per mile; someone weighing 120 pounds, 80 calories per mile.

START EXERCISING
BEFORE YOU QUIT

If you've been sedentary for a long time, first see your doctor for the go-ahead, and then when you're ready, preferably a month before your quit day, start exercising slowly. Begin with a short walk at a comfortable pace—slightly above a stroll—for 10 to 15 minutes, three times a week. This should burn between 150 and 225 calories per week. As you near your quit date, increase your walking to two miles a day, five days a week, so that you are burning off about 1,000 calories per week. This alone may be enough to offset the anticipated 200-calorie-per-day decrease in your metabolism. If you avoid overeating, you shouldn't gain weight after quitting smoking.

If your goal is to *lose* weight, continue to build up the walking until you're burning between 1,500 and 2,000 calories per week. If you walk 20 miles each week, you'll be using up an extra 2,000 calories or so. That breaks down to about three miles per day, or a one-hour walk seven days a week. That's a great goal, regardless of your weight. It may sound like a lot of walking, but remember that you don't have to do it all at once. Walking 30 minutes in the morning and 30 minutes at night is a good way to break it up.

The chart below shows you how easy it is to burn 200 calories through a variety of physical activities. The calculations are based on a 150-pound person; if you weigh more, then it will take you less time to burn 200 calories and if you weigh less, it will take slightly longer. To prevent weight gain, try to get at least 30 minutes (or 200 calories expended) of moderate exercise or, better still, endurance-type activity (see page 111) on most—preferably all—days of the week.

PHYSICAL ACTIVITY	TIME REQUIRED
Bicycling 4 miles	20 minutes
Jumping rope	20 minutes
Running 1.5 miles (10 min./mile)	20 minutes
Shoveling snow	20 minutes
Stairwalking	20 minutes
Basketball (playing game)	20–25 minutes
Swimming laps	25 minutes
Dancing fast	30 minutes
Basketball (shooting baskets)	40 minutes
Bicycling 5 miles	40 minutes
Raking leaves	40 minutes
Walking 2 miles (20 min./mile)	40 minutes
Water aerobics	40 minutes
Wheeling self in wheelchair	40–55 minutes
Gardening	40–60 minutes
Playing touch football	40–60 minutes
Walking 1.75 miles (20 min./mile)	45 minutes
Playing volleyball	60 minutes
Washing and waxing car	60–80 minutes
Washing windows or floor	60–80 minutes

THE NEXT LEVEL OF FITNESS

When choosing an exercise program, aim to keep a balance between the following three equally important elements.

1. Cardiovascular workouts utilize your large muscles to burn calories and increase your heart rate. Try to do three to five sessions of 20 to 45 minutes weekly. Examples of this type of workout include brisk walking, jogging, bicycling, spinning (the newest fad for cyclists), box aerobics classes, cross-country ski machines, swimming, aerobic dance classes, and stair climbing.

2. Strength training is based on using resistance weights, machines, and/or elastic bands to strengthen and shape your muscles. Aim for two to three sessions weekly and include at least one exercise for every major muscle group—buttocks, legs, back, chest, arms, and abdomen. These can be done with free weights or machine weights. Many gyms offer body-sculpting classes or workouts with free weights.

3. Flexibility exercises loosen your muscles and relax your mind. Ideally, you should stretch at the beginning of each session or after 10 minutes or so of walking or light jogging, and again at the end of the session. Stretching purports to help avoid injury, but if not done properly, it can actually cause problems. Be especially careful if you exercise in the morning when your muscles, ligaments, and tendons are like rubber bands kept in a refrigerator overnight—too much stretching can cause them to tear. To avoid this, do gentle stretches or simply begin your chosen exercise for about 10 minutes to warm yourself up, then stop and do more intense stretching. Some people prefer to stretch at the end of a session, which is not ideal but will improve flexibility nonetheless. Always stretch your calves, ankles, shoulders, and back for 5 to 10 minutes as part of your routine.

Choose the exercise program that best reduces your stress level as well. While some people find that walking or running every day gives them an endorphin high and a sense of well-being, others may think it adds to the driving force of the day, resulting in more, not less, stress. Understand who you are and how you work. If you already feel as if you're on a treadmill, a slower pace might be exactly what you need. Try integrating disciplines that focus on one movement at a time, such as Pilates or yoga, into your life.

If, however, you love having an all-out 400-calorie burn and find that it helps to clear your mind, plan to fit it in once or twice a week. On other days, especially if you've been cooped in all day, try walking around the block four or five times. This will help you get fresh air, relieve stress, and add a measure of satisfaction to your day. The key is reading yourself, figuring out what you like, and finding ways to fit the activity into your day. If you stress out about your exercise program, you won't be as consistent with it. Do what works for you and your lifestyle.

AN EXAMPLE FOR EVERYONE

Here's a textbook example of how to integrate regular exercise into your life. It's not based on a health nut or a model, but on a man with an average body and a normal life with normal stresses. You'll learn from him, be inspired by him, and most of all, relate to him.

Gary is a 48-year-old Hollywood movie producer, married with two great children, who finally seemed to be on the winning side of his smoking and weight battle. He had stopped smoking several times, once for two years, but always started again. Although he could stay off cigarettes in between movie projects, he would start smoking again as soon as the cameras rolled. Then a friend of his had a heart attack and Gary was scared into quitting for good.

Since he had been through quitting a number of times, Gary knew the routine. At 6 feet 1 inch tall, his ideal weight was 175 pounds. When he stopped smoking, he put on 15 pounds in six months, only to lose the weight when he picked up cigarettes again. But this time when he quit for good, he found a way to keep the weight off.

The Workout

Gary was committed to doing a brisk 50-minute walk on his treadmill two times a week, and whenever he could, he added two or three 20-minute walks, also usually on the treadmill. If he had a late afternoon appointment, for example, Gary would get on the treadmill at 3:00 P.M. for a quick 20 minutes before he ran out the door. He found that this burst of activity was enough to keep his stress down *and* his weight in check without resorting to smoking.

Gary spent a lot of time each day on the phone. He realized that he could utilize this downtime and burn an average of 100 to 150 calories more each day just by purchasing a headphone set for the telephone: Now he could walk while he talked. This activity also helped distract him from his usual urge to light up while on the phone.

On weekends, Gary spent about 30 minutes daily lifting weights at a gym. He devised a routine with his trainer that included over-the-head presses to strengthen his shoulders, and a variation of curls and lateral flies to build up his biceps. Since he wanted to work out at home as well, he purchased 5-, 8-, 10-, 12-, 15-, and 20-pound weights. (See page 114 for tips on buying weights.)

The Diet

Gary started his day with a cup of coffee and a big bowl of oatmeal. Besides helping to lower his blood cholesterol levels, the oatmeal had a "stick to the ribs" quality that helped him eat a sensible lunch. His lunch would be a salad and pasta, or fish or chicken with a small portion of rice or pasta, and he generally ate only about three-quarters of what was on his plate. One of his guiding philosophies was, "Don't eat it unless you *really* like it." Gary found he could indulge in his favorite chicken burritos with beans and salsa if he skipped the chips, cheese, guacamole, and sour cream, garnishes that only added extra fat and calories. He also learned to enjoy one of his stand-by lunches, kung pao shrimp, with just a half cup of rice. Gary ate nuts for snacks—knowing that they had all the protein, fat, and carbohydrates he needed to tide him over to the next meal—and made sure to keep his portions to a handful. (Nuts contain about 200 calories per ¼ cup—a good amount for a snack.)

The Written Record

Gary sums up his weight-management secret in three words: "Write everything down." He has kept records of his food and exercise regimens for the last three years, and even though his routine has become a way of life, he thinks this is paramount to keeping him on track.

You too should log your daily exercise in your food and exercise diary. If you want, take the number of calories you burn during exercise and subtract that figure from your food intake for an adjusted value. After two weeks, you'll know how many calories your body really needs to maintain or achieve a certain weight—then you can work toward that goal on a daily basis. If you overeat one day, you can make it up the next day by eating less and perhaps exercising more. Just avoiding fasting or a severe restriction of food intake to prevent bingeing later on. Remember, when it comes to food, a little effort over a long period of time is much better than a big effort that doesn't last.

WEIGHT TRAINING

Anaerobic exercise, such as weight training, also benefits new ex-smokers who have been inactive for some time. Brief and frequent weight-lifting sessions increase lean body mass or muscle, which in turn boosts your metabolism and the calories you expend each day. An ideal lean-to-fat ratio, or body composition, is essential to overall fitness and optimal weight management. An effective strength-training routine consists of lifting one weight 8 to 10 times for every five major muscle groups. It may take only 10 to 15 minutes every other day to increase lean body mass, strength, and bone density. You don't even need to go to a gym. Just purchase a few weights that you can work with at home.

BUYING WEIGHTS

According to Leslie Goetzman, a personal trainer and exercise physiologist, women generally start with 2-, 5-, and 8-pound weights and eventually, after a few solid months of training, go on to 15-pound weights. Men typically start with 5-, 8-, 10-, 12-, 15-, and 20-pound weights. Weights vary in price from roughly 69¢ a pound to as much as $3 a pound. Chrome weights are at the upper end of the price range (they're nice because they don't chip), and iron and lead weights are at the lower end. (Avoid lead if you have children who may put them in their mouths.) Some weights have a neoprene covering—the material wet suits are made of—which gives them a comfortable grip. You can even use soup cans if you don't want to spend money on weights.

If you'd rather stretch than lift, try elastic exercise bands. An alternative to weights as a source of resistance, they are a preferable method for people who have joint problems. The resistance is consistent so the technique and strength required is more even through the range of motion in a typical workout. They're also lightweight, and especially convenient to throw in your suitcase when you travel.

CHAPTER 8
Smart Snacking
That Satisfies

Snacks can help. It's that simple. During this stressful time, when you've just quit smoking and are getting over your nicotine addiction, you'll probably be tempted to reach for a snack instead of a cigarette. You know what snacks are: little in-between bites, like a handful of chips, a few cookies, a taste from last night's leftovers, even a piece of fruit. But not all snacks are healthy, though it's wise to remember that any food you put in your mouth is bound to be healthier than a cigarette. This chapter's goal is to help you learn how to snack *smart*, without overloading on calories in the process. It's a balance, but you can do it.

SNACK TO FEEL SATISFIED—
AND EAT FEWER CALORIES

How can you replace tobacco with snacks and still control your weight? The trick is to stay within your overall calorie limit, which you determined in Chapter 5, and to choose those foods that will give you an edge—i.e., that feeling of fullness, without a calorie overload. Remember one important point: Low-fat foods contain calories, too. Weight management is not just a matter of cutting out fat, or replacing high-fat foods with low-fat foods. If you snack on low-fat foods that are still high in calories, like fat-free pretzels, cookies, or chips, you may be getting many more calories than you need.

But there is a smart snacking solution, according to Barbara Rolls, Ph.D., professor of nutrition at Penn State University. As she outlines in her book, *Volumetrics* (New York: HarperCollins, 2000), most people eat a constant *weight* of food each day, regardless of the food's fat content. If you focus on the *quantity* of foods you eat that are packed with water or fiber but not calories, such as fruits, vegetables, and grains, you're likely to feel just as full as if you ate the same amount of high-fat, high-calorie foods. The difference is that you'll be getting a fraction of the fat and calories!

This corresponds with the style of eating discussed in Chapter 4—a diet of whole grains, fruits, vegetables, beans, nonfat or low-fat dairy products, lean beef, poultry, and fish. Lowering your calorie intake can be as simple as choosing more fruits and vegetables as snacks. If you apply these guidelines to snacks as well as meals, you'll have a new assortment of foods to reach for when the craving strikes: smart snacks.

Fresh fruits are lower in calorie density than dried fruits; a quarter cup of raisins is calorically equal to nearly two cups of grapes, for example. Smoothies (see page 16) made with yogurt, ice, banana, an orange, and a little honey or sugar, are another sensible, nutrient-packed choice. Ounce for ounce, high-fiber cereals are calorically lower than sugary, low-fiber cereals, so eat oatmeal or bran flakes instead of Fruit Loops and Sugar Pops. Nonfat or low-fat milk is also a good bet, as most of its weight is water, not to mention the protein, calcium, and vitamin D it packs.

When choosing a snack, check the calories, the fiber content, and the portion size. If the calories are high and the portion size is small, find another option. Low-calorie, high-fiber foods are emptied from the stomach more slowly and take longer to digest, giving your brain a full feeling for a longer period of time, which helps tide you over to the next meal. If you're confronting a serious nicotine craving, you're better off choosing dense low-calorie foods like carrots, for example, because they're harder to overeat. You can even include some higher-fat and higher-calorie foods if you watch the portion sizes. You'll find suggested portion sizes in the lists on page 128. What's exciting is that there really are ways to eat fewer calories and not feel hungry.

Snacking can actually benefit your overall health if you choose wisely and use some restraint. Here are the eight rules of smart snacking.

1. Select foods that provide a large volume compared to their calorie level.

HERE'S WHY: As explained above, a large volume of low-calorie foods will leave you with the same level of fullness as a large volume of high-calorie foods. Since it's really the amount of food we eat that determines fullness, it's easy to choose foods that don't have such a negative effect on our weight—and still feel satisfied.

For example, let's compare an apple with a chocolate chip cookie. An apple weighs about five ounces and has 80 calories. A chocolate chip cookie weighs about an ounce—one-fifth the apple's weight—yet has 160 calories, or twice that of the apple! (Incidentally, a reduced-fat chocolate chip cookie still has 150 calories!) Fiber and water lower the calories in food; fat has the opposite effect. The apple, like most fruits and vegetables, is not only low in fat but full of fiber and water, as well. The cookie, by contrast, has little water or moisture but plenty of refined flour and sugar. Even fat-free and sugar-free foods like pretzels can be surprisingly calorie-dense. "Since they have little fiber or water, you can take in a lot of calories while you think you're not eating that much," says Barbara Rolls.

HERE'S HOW: So should you always opt for the apple instead of the cookie? Not necessarily. As you learned in the chapter about cravings, you may be more satisfied with a cookie than with an apple. Instead of eating a handful, however, try just one or two cookies along with a glass of nonfat milk. That way, you'll have consumed a filling snack with fewer calories than if you just ate the cookies alone. Consider choosing low-calorie cookies too, since cutting back on the fat will not affect the weight of the cookie—and a low-fat cookie should fill you up just as well.

2. Use snacking to avoid weight gain.

HERE'S WHY: When you stop smoking, your appetite often increases (see page 9). Used properly, snacking can cut down on the size of your meals, particularly lunch and dinner, and in this way help prevent weight gain. Reaching for some yogurt, fruit, or even a sweet may control your hunger and help you avoid overeating at mealtimes. The key is to eat the right amount of the right snack in between small meals. Not only does this keep you from overeating, it also keeps your metabolic rate higher than if you ate less frequently. A higher metabolism means you're burning more calories.

HERE'S HOW: The idea, of course, is not to fill up but to snack just enough so that by lunch or dinner you are in control of your choices, not swayed by a rumbling stomach. Keep snacks light so that the snack-plus-meal combination does not lead to calorie overload, not to mention the sluggish feeling that comes with it. Snacks should equal 25 percent of your total daily caloric intake, with the remaining 75 percent derived from breakfast, lunch, and dinner. If you need 1,600 calories a day, you should get about 400 calories from snacks. Refer to the calorie requirement guidelines in Chapter 5 on page 70 to determine your calorie limit.

Keep healthy snacks on hand in your purse or briefcase, or in the refrigerator at your office. Being prepared with an apple, orange, cookie, or some crackers with cheese or peanut butter will help you respond to hunger signals. See the list of snacks on page 127 for more ideas. Make a mental note of when you ate your last meal, and never go more than five hours until the next one, at least not without a snack in between.

3. Get in touch with what you really want to snack on.

HERE'S WHY: As explained in Chapter 3 on cravings, there may be a biological basis for the food you desire. If you go right for your target food, you'll feel better with a small amount.

HERE'S HOW: If it's a sweet you crave, fruit may not do; satisfy your sweet tooth with frozen yogurt, a cookie and milk, or sweetened cereal. If it's chocolate you crave, have a small portion. Try four chocolate kisses for 100 calories. Couple your treat with a hot beverage such as herb tea, decaffeinated coffee, or sugar-free or low-fat cocoa. This way, chocolate doesn't take center stage. A beverage also helps to get the sweet taste out of your mouth, because if it stays there you're likely to want more. You may want to try brushing your teeth as well. Check the list of snacks on page 127 to find the calorie level that will meet your needs.

4. Use snacking for a nutritional boost.

HERE'S WHY: Part of the wisdom of hunger is to ensure that the body meets its needs for vitamins, minerals, and fiber. Keep in mind that snacking can satisfy nutritional gaps as well as control a raging appetite. Munching on a red bell pepper, for example, will boost your vitamin C level to 130 percent and your vitamin A level to 15 percent of the U.S. RDA. Many of my clients claim they don't have time to snack on nutritious food, but a lot of smart snacks take less time to prepare than starting the car or grabbing a candy bar from a vending machine. The only thing you have to remember is to bring them along with you!

HERE'S HOW: In the morning, reach for fruit or yogurt rather than baked goods. Then choose your snack according to when you expect to eat next. A pure carbohydrate snack such as fruit or bread is digested and absorbed within 30 to 60 minutes, so it gives you fast energy. But you'll get hungry again, quickly. That's okay if the next meal is around the corner. For maximum satiation, choose a snack that combines carbohydrates, protein, and fat, such as peanut butter on apple slices or a cracker with low-fat cheese.

5. When it's sweets you crave, remember moderation.

HERE'S WHY: Sugar belongs in your life, but let's give it a proper place. While a small dose of a sugary food can ease your cravings and calm you down, a large amount can ultimately have the opposite effect.

According to Janet Lepke, R.D., C.D.E., L.D.N., owner of Nutrition Network in Charlotte, North Carolina, sweets cannot bear the full responsibility for treating your stress. "It's like relieving a headache with pain medication," she says. "You only need one pain pill, and then you also need to relax, take a hot bath, have a cup of tea. Think of sugar as a privilege that you don't want to abuse. Like the plumber who doesn't take your wedding pictures, sugar can't solve all your problems."

HERE'S HOW: Lepke suggests: "If you have a yen for sugar, try chewing gummy bears or licorice because they are actually low in sugar as well as calories. And since they take longer to chew, you're less likely to get through an entire bag of gummy bears than cookies, for example. All this chewing can be helpful—it may also soothe the frustration and anger you may be feeling."

6. Avoid overeating healthy foods.

HERE'S WHY: Many health-conscious snackers over-snack on what are considered "good" foods: cereal, crackers, whole-grain bread, and bagels. That may be an improvement over high-fat chips and cookies, but the excessive calories in these foods still get stored as fat, even if they are otherwise healthy calories. Some people overeat fruit or drink large amounts of fruit juice, especially in the summer when fruits are in season and taste so good. Fruits remain a great snack, but remember that they do contain calories.

HERE'S HOW: Figure out how many calories you burn per day by using the chart on page 70, then keep track of the foods you eat and add up the day's calories. Be sure to subtract exercise calories. The results may help you control snacking a bit more. Also try eating more vegetables as snacks—remember, you should get five servings of fruit and/or vegetables each day. If you like to eat a larger volume of food, eat more of low-calorie vegetables such as salad greens, bell peppers, summer squash, and broccoli. Alternatively, choose soup. According to Barbara Rolls, soup is the dieter's secret weapon, especially broth-based, vegetable types that contain a lot of water and fiber with relatively few calories. Finally, go for fresh fruit rather than fruit juice most of the time. If you do have juice, keep the portion to four to eight ounces.

7. Avoid mindless snacking.

HERE'S WHY: Calories add up when you take a bite of this and spoonful of that while you're cooking, watching TV, or making small talk at a cocktail party. It's too easy for a cookie or two to turn into a whole bag of cookies.

HERE'S HOW: Have a snack only when you're hungry or craving a particular food. Eat consciously; experience and savor the food as you're eating it. Portion out your snacks rather than eat them from a bag. Better yet, choose preportioned snacks, such as frozen juice bars, reduced-fat ice cream bars, or granola bars. Don't cue your hunger by leaving snacks on the counter or anywhere in sight.

If it's oral stimulation you crave, try a nonfood substitute or a food that takes some "work," such as unshelled sunflower seeds. Dr. Keith Pendell, who conducts smoking cessation training sessions for people who work with teens, warns against eating too much to compensate for quitting cigarettes. "Snacking is one thing," he says, "but if you are merely substituting one addiction for another, it will catch up with you." Dr. Pendell has a number of substitutes he recommends to his clients when they need to put something in their mouths. His list includes:

- toothpicks
- sunflower seeds (unshelled)
- hard candy
- sugar-free chewing gum
- plastic straws
- plastic coffee stirrers
- cinnamon sticks

And if keeping your hands occupied is a problem, try manipulating an item like a pencil or a small rubber ball. Here are a few additional non-oral substitutes:

- silly putty
- golf pencil and doodle paper
- rubber band around your wrist—snap it when you're tempted to smoke or eat when you're not hungry!

8. Identify Your Irresistible Foods.

HERE'S WHY: We all have one or two foods that are in the category of "Don't *even* get me started." These are called trigger foods because they set off a path of overeating that's hard to stop. As important as it is to eat occasional treats, it's also important to accept that there will never be a time when you can eat whatever you want, whenever you want.

HERE'S HOW: Rather than giving up trigger foods completely, learn to eat them in controlled situations. One of my clients, Marie, had an irresistible weakness for chocolate chip cookies. "If there was a bag of cookies in my pantry, I'd hear them calling my name," she explained. As a way to monitor her trigger food binges, she decided to eat her favorite cookie only when she was away from home at coffee bars, restaurants, or a friend's apartment. She discovered that she could control her cravings much more easily if she ate with other people around, and on these special occasions, she limited herself to one cookie only. Marie also began to shop at supermarkets that sold individual cookies so she could avoid buying a box of cookies. She discovered that it was much easier to say no to a single supermarket cookie than to ignore an entire bag calling out her name from the pantry.

Make a list of your own trigger foods and keep it with you when you shop. You don't have to stop eating your favorite foods—just make sure that you control your indulgences, not the other way around.

SMART SNACKING ON THE GO

When you smoked, you probably always carried cigarettes with you, right? Why not do the same for snacks? Pack an apple or a banana and a bottle of water before you go out—toss them into your purse or your car—and you're set. You won't forget them any more than you'd forget your cigarettes in the old days. Even if you don't end up eating the food, it's there if you want it. This is a preventive measure to help you resist those vending machines at work or school, which can be tempting. Vending machine choices, though improving, are still largely limited to chips, cookies, and candy bars, with an occasional bag of peanuts.

SMART SNACKING AT MEETINGS AND PARTIES

Meeting the challenge of staying smoke-free at a party could come at the price of overeating. Don't let it. Limit high-calorie, high-fat foods at social situations. Ask yourself this question *ahead of time:* Will I let these appetizers whet my appetite, or will they become my dinner? It's okay to replace dinner with happy hour or snacks, as long as you make the right choices. Stock up on vegetables, go easy on high-fat dips, and use a limited amount of cheese on plain crackers and bread. Subject your food to the grease test—if it spreads a ring of grease on your napkin, forget it.

You can enjoy yourself without depending on huge quantities of food to make the event pleasant. Find someone interesting to talk to; be an interesting person to talk to. And position yourself away from the food when you're at a meeting or cocktail party.

SMART SNACKING AT SPORTING EVENTS AND MOVIES

These situations set you up to snack, not to mention smoke. Richard, one of my clients, is a longtime hockey fan and has season tickets to the Los Angeles games, which means he goes three or four nights a week when the team is at home. Richard is the president of his own advertising agency, and does everything he can to finish on time on game days so he can be there for the start of the game. Arriving hungry and all wound up from a tense day, he usually drinks a beer, eats a hot dog, has popcorn, and then ice cream. These game-day meals add up to about 1,500 calories, nearly 50 percent of which are fat!

Richard asks me, "Is this okay?" In view of the fact that he's trying to take off the 30 pounds he put on since he quit smoking last year, that he is 41 years old with a family and a wonderful future ahead of him, and that his father died of heart disease at a young age, the answer is no. Richard is heading in the wrong direction fast.

I advised Richard, as I have many other clients, to eat *before* going to the game. His solution was to pick up a chicken burrito with rice and beans from the local Rotisserie Chicken drive-through, and eat it at the game. If he had to order food at the game, we decided it should be one or two items instead of three or four, and preferably lower-fat choices such as a turkey sandwich, a hot pretzel, or popcorn.

LATE-NIGHT SMART SNACKING

Besides being a nutritional nightmare, one of the chief culprits in weight gain is out-of-control late night snacking. There are three big problems with late night snacking: too many calories, poor sleep, and a tendency to skip breakfast—and the cycle tends to repeat itself the next day. According to Dr. Anthony Reading, clinical psychologist and professor at the University of California, Los Angeles, people often eat when they are overtired and fatigued. "When you're sleep-deprived," he says, "you can't meet the intellectual challenge of making decisions, so you take the line of least resistance and do something you *can* do—eat."

Dr. Reading says that overeating at night is often linked with the following:

1. Insomnia
2. Worry
3. Insufficient eating during the day
4. Lack of fulfillment or satisfaction (i.e., your day is ending and you sense a lack of harmony or balance)
5. The feeling of being revved up or turned on by internal physiology (i.e., just when you should be winding down, you're getting your second wind)
6. Isolation, emptiness, the need for solace—an alternative to saying prayers
7. Repressed, expressed, or partially expressed sexual energy

This is a long list and some of the underlying factors are not easy to solve. Begin by making a conscious transition from your daytime to your evening mode. "Don't expect to go from a hectic pace during the day to a relaxed mode at night without allowing some transition time," says Dr. Reading. "Start by eating three regular meals in the daytime so you can quell the urge to snack at night. Plan something, such as gardening or cooking, to help you make the transition."

If you do snack, *stop snacking within an hour or two of bedtime.* Dr. Reading suggests that if feelings of isolation are the source of snacking, try engaging others in conversation. Some people are finding new outlets through the Internet, where they can connect with other people in virtual chat rooms. This can be very helpful. Another tactic is to delay and distract: Wait 5 or 10 minutes and the urge to eat may pass, or distract yourself with a phone call, a bath, or a walk around the block. If you still need to eat something, it's probably a craving. You'll find lots of ways to deal with cravings in Chapter 3.

BEWARE OF TELEVISION'S INFLUENCE

It's been said that God is in the minutia and the devil is in the television. According to Dr. Reading, "TV provides some people with nervous stimulation—it jiggles you up without any real fulfillment. You are understimulated in a real way like the taste that never satisfies, making you feel insecure, dissatisfied, and dejected—all the things you don't want, so you reach for the cookie jar."

Television also influences your eating patterns in another way. During an average hour of prime-time TV, you probably watch eight or nine commercials for food products. At the same time, many of the actresses touting those products maintain amazingly low body weights. According to nutritionist Janet Lepke, "When you see the completely unrealistic portrayal of an actress eating a piece of apple pie á la mode while she's wearing her midriff top with belly button exposed, it's an impossible standard to meet. You're getting one message to eat ice cream and apple pie and another to be very thin."

Remember that snacking, not to mention late night cravings, is normal. If you're smart and use the information in this chapter, you'll find your way. Quitting smoking is one of the hardest things you'll do in your life, but you can do it—without gaining weight.

THE PERSONAL NUTRITION MANAGEMENT PLAN FOR SMART SNACKS

Eat the *right* snacks and you'll meet your calorie needs without sacrificing good nutrition. The Personal Nutrition Management Plan for Smart Snacks is designed to be an eating style you will stay with for the long term. Use the list below to select foods with the best caloric value for your ultimate snacking satisfaction. When appropriate check food-package labels for calorie values. Be sure to log them into your food journal and stay within your calorie limit.

25 CALORIES OR LESS

VEGETABLES

Artichoke (½ medium)
Artichoke hearts (¼ cup)
Asparagus (6 spears)
Broccoli (½ cup)
Cabbage (½ cup)
Carrots (1 medium)
Cauliflower (½ cup)
Celery (4 stalks)
Crunchy Cucumber Slices
  (page 190) (½ cup)
Cucumber (½ cup)
Eggplant (½ cup)
Peppers, all varieties (½ cup)
Radishes (10 medium)
Salad greens (1 cup)
Sauerkraut (½ cup)
Snow Peas (½ cup)
Summer squash (½ cup)
Tomato (1 medium)
Tomato/vegetable juice (½ cup)
Zucchini (½ cup)

SUGAR-FREE OR LOW-SUGAR FOODS

Candy, hard, sugar-free (2 pieces)
Gelatin dessert, sugar-free (1 cup)
Jam or jelly, low-sugar or light (2
  tablespoons)

DRINKS

Bouillon, broth, or consommé
Carbonated or mineral water
Coffee
Club soda
Diet soft drinks, sugar-free

MISCELLANEOUS

Olives, green (4)
Pickles, dill (1 large)

100 CALORIES OR LESS

FRUITS AND VEGETABLES

Apple, Banana, Oranges

Apple, Cucumber, and Cilantro Salad

Carrot Juice

Celery with Cottage Cheese

Melon Popsicles (page 271)

Pureed vegetable soup

Raw Mushroom Sandwich

Sautéed Zucchini with Garlic
(page 260)

Thin Turkey Breast Slices with Melon

DAIRY

Yogurt Cone

SWEETS AND STARCHES

Bagel Crisp with Mozzarella
Cheese

Baked Potato Chips

Chewy Brownies (page 266)

Chocolate chips

Chocolate kisses

Crunchy Oatmeal Chocolate Chip
Cookie (page 274)

Fig Newtons

Forget-Me-Not Meringue
(page 273)

Ginger Snaps

200 CALORIES OR LESS

FRUIT

Apple and Low-fat Cheddar Cheese

Banana with Peanut Butter

Chicken Salad with Apple
(page 186)

Chinese Chicken Salad (page 187)

Fruit salad with Wheat Germ

Gazpacho (page 175)

Mango and Cottage Cheese

DAIRY

Chocolate Pudding (page 269)

Easy Frozen Strawberry-Banana Pie
(page 275)

Light ice cream or frozen yogurt

SWEETS AND STARCHES

Baked Sweet Potato

Baked Garlic Fries and ketchup
(page 248)

Barbecued Chicken Pizza (page 229)

Bran Flakes

Crunchy Granola with milk
(page 157)

Easy Ham and Cheese Quesadilla
(page 247)

English Muffin with butter or
margarine or jam

Graham crackers and 1% milk

Hard-boiled Eggs and Wasa Crackers

200 CALORIES OR LESS
(cont.)

SWEETS AND STARCHES

Low-fat cereals with milk

1% Cottage Cheese and sliced
   strawberries on ½ English
   Muffin

Pita with Ham and Tomato

Pretzels

Refrigerator Buttermilk Bran
   Muffin (page 164)

MAKING IT HAPPEN

Consider it your goal to eat healthier snacks in the appropriate amounts. Use
this system to make it happen:

1. Put your snack choices on your shopping list.
2. Shop at least once a week and buy most of your food for the
week, including fresh vegetables.
3. Prepare cut-up vegetables and fruit either before you put them
away or when you are making a salad at dinnertime. Also prepare a
few extra vegetables for the next day or two. If you know you
won't go to the fuss, buy packaged pre-prepped vegetables from
your supermarket.

CHAPTER 9
Dining Out Tips

Let's face it, everyone likes to eat. Food is one of life's great pleasures, and there is no reason why anyone should have to live without the gratification that comes from enjoying a delicious, well-prepared meal. Often, restaurant food is even tastier than the food you cook at home; after all, chefs are trained professionals. In the previous chapters of this book, you learned how to make sensible choices about what to eat so that after quitting smoking, you can avoid replacing that bad habit with a tendency to eat too much high-fat, high-calorie food. It's easy to follow a healthy regime at home, where you have nutrition labels and calorie charts to help you calculate your meals for the day. Unfortunately, counting calories and fat grams is not as easy to do at restaurants.

If you are like many Americans today, dining out is one of your favorite hobbies. But because of the way restaurant food is served, and depending on how often you eat out, restaurant dining can shoot down your entire weight-watching strategy. Whether you dine out four times a week or once a month, you'll need to fit restaurant choices into your new, healthier, tobacco-free lifestyle.

For the recovering ex-smoker, a restaurant may encourage your former bad habit, but you can avoid temptation. Ask to be seated in the nonsmoking section. Depending on what type of smoker you are (see Chapter 2 to help evaluate your habits), look for some physical and/or mental activity that will take the place of smoking. It may be something to involve your hands and mouth, like chewing on a toothpick, or it might be something to occupy your mind, like composing a poem on a paper napkin. Now turn to the issue of food: Many people think they can't dine out and still eat healthfully, but that's simply not true.

There are two keys to incorporating restaurant dining into a healthy lifestyle. First, you must order foods that will fall within your calorie and fat limits. Second, you must find a realistic way to deal with the gargantuan portion sizes you're likely to encounter.

WHAT TO ORDER

Restaurant chefs don't have anyone looking over their shoulder telling them to lighten up, so they don't. Fat is the lazy cook's route to flavor—making food taste delicious without fat takes time, effort, and expense. Most restaurants take the easy way out. The best strategy when dining out is to order plain foods, without sauce, and those dishes that require very little fat in order to taste good—or none at all. Sushi, pork fajitas, and fruit sorbet are a few examples.

Order simple foods because it's hard to tell what's in certain dishes, especially those that combine a lot of ingredients. Most calories and fat are "hidden" so you don't know what you're getting. Was the pizza topped with a half cup or two cups of cheese? Is there a tablespoon of oil in your pasta sauce or is a quarter cup more like it? Always choose the simpler item on the menu: a baked potato rather than mashed potatoes; plain grilled chicken or fish rather than one in a heavy sauce. Avoid adding butter to bread or rolls—or just skip the bread. You will almost certainly get enough calories from your entrée by itself. If you eat out frequently and have consistently large portions with more fat than you're counting on, you're likely to experience a significant rise in your weight. This calls for exercising portion control.

DEALING WITH
RESTAURANT PORTIONS

Trying to estimate how many calories, carbohydrate, and fat grams are in your restaurant meal is perhaps the greatest challenge of dining away from home. You've probably noticed a trend in the restaurant world toward bigger and bigger portions, and it's tricky to guess how much food is on your plate.

Deciding whether you're eating two or three cups of spaghetti can represent a difference of 250 calories, or even more.

Since calories have the greatest bearing on your weight, it's crucial to pay attention to portion size. Remember that a huge gap exists between the amount of calories you eat at home and the amount you're likely to be served at a restaurant. When dining at home, a typical dinner serving might include 1½ cups of pasta and ½ cup of sauce for 350 to 400 calories. But restaurants typically serve 2½ cups of pasta, not to mention the sauce, and that's likely to add up to 800 calories!

Restaurant dishes like pasta can still fit into your plan, but only if you eat them in smaller quantities. Consuming large amounts of high-carbohydrate foods will make your calorie count go sky high, and that means probable weight gain. Unfortunately, carbohydrates like pasta, bread, and bagels are very easy to overeat—who hasn't been seduced by the bottomless bread basket?

Whatever you order, keep in mind that a restaurant meal with all the trimmings is likely to be double your calorie needs. Start with ordering less. The other logical strategy is to not eat everything on your plate. That may be a departure from your normal way of dining, and it takes some practice but can be done. Use this tactic when the food tastes so delicious that you want to finish it, or when you're out with family or friends, perhaps having a glass of wine and a jolly time, your inhibitions are down, and you are more likely to overeat. Here are 10 additional tips that can help you control your food intake when you dine out. Practice them until they become habits.

1. Check the list of appetizers. You may find one or two that will satisfy you as an entrée.
2. Order appetizer portions of an entrée.
3. Order salad and soup, or perhaps just one or the other if the serving size is large enough. Ask for salad dressing on the side so you can add only as much as you want.
4. Pasta is a risky meal to order in a restaurant, so proceed with caution. It's best to order a half portion or an appetizer portion. If neither is available, eat half and take the other half home. Even if it has a low-fat sauce, it's important to limit the amount of pasta itself. Avoid dishes with cream sauce.

5. Share an entrée with a friend.

6. Pass on the bread. If you can't control yourself, set it out of your reach or ask the waiter to take it away.

7. As soon as you're finished with half of your meal, ask your server to take your plate. Consider taking the rest home for lunch the next day.

8. After a meal in which you've stayed within your limits, remind yourself of how good you feel. When you've eaten to the point that you're uncomfortable, be very conscious of that feeling and notice how it isn't much fun to feel stuffed. Instead of flogging yourself and feeling guilty, just make up your mind to do it differently next time.

9. If you plan to have dessert, you should probably skip both the bread and the rice, potatoes, or pasta. Instead, order a nice plate of sautéed vegetables with your protein.

10. Control your alcohol intake; follow any guidelines provided by your doctor. Alcohol adds extra calories and stimulates the appetite while simultaneously decreasing your inhibitions: just what you don't need in a restaurant situation.

Remember, it's not a good idea to overeat at a restaurant, even if it's a special occasion. Most Americans dine out an average of four times a week, according to Hope Warshaw, M.M.Sc., R.D., C.D.E., author of *The Restaurant Companion, a Guide to Healthier Eating Out* (Chicago: Surrey Books, 1995). As she points out, "It will be difficult to achieve your health and nutrition goals if there's always an opportunity to overeat." Warshaw's book offers tips on ordering healthful meals from Mexican, Chinese, Italian, Thai, Indian, and Middle Eastern cuisines, and even includes fast food restaurants with calorie values from many of their menus. This valuable resource can help you make the best selections when dining out. You may also want to check the food values listed in the appendix of this book.

WRESTLING WITH THE FOOD PYRAMID

If you use the U.S.D.A. Food Guide Pyramid to help keep track of your healthy dining habits, be aware of one thing. Lisa Young, a registered dietitian who has run weight-loss programs and is currently a doctoral candidate at New York University, is writing her dissertation on portion size. According to Lisa Young, many foods on the Pyramid are measured in "cocktail" servings, but in real life everything from bagels to restaurant entrées is getting larger. Because the serving sizes on the Pyramid (as they're defined on the nutrition label) may be smaller than what you actually eat, you must rework the math. The Pyramid considers a serving of meat as 2 to 3 ounces, but eating 2 ounces of meat is not particularly common—when was the last time you saw a 2-ounce steak? If you regularly eat 4 ounces of meat—think of a quarter-pound hamburger—you must count it as two servings. Similarly, a Pyramid serving of cereal is half a cup, but if you tend to eat 1 cup at breakfast it counts as two servings.

Now consider the baked potato in the Food Guide Pyramid: It's calculated as 3 ounces at 80 calories. But a potato of that size would never be served at a restaurant; a more typical potato is 6 to 8 ounces with anywhere from 160 to 240 calories, easily two or three carbohydrate servings. At some restaurants, particularly steak houses, a baked potato might even tip the scale at 10 or 12 ounces. Here's a good test: The next time you're in a supermarket, weigh a few potatoes of different sizes. That way, you'll get better at eyeballing restaurant portions and can leave the part of the potato that's too big for your meal plan (or even better, doggie bag it). Also get to know what 3 ounces of meat looks like (about the size of a pack of cards).

Be a more accurate judge of how much food you are consuming and fit it into your optimum daily meal plan. Look at the guide on page 71 to determine how many calories you need throughout the day. Most important, become familiar with the calorie values of various foods so you can determine how a restaurant meal fits into your particular plan. Sound complicated? After a few trips to the supermarket scale with your favorite foods, you'll become an expert at eyeballing.

NUTS AND BOLTS: SMART ORDERING ADVICE FOR RESTAURANT DINING

Breakfast

YES

- Cold Cereal (Whole-Grain or Shredded Wheat with Nonfat or Low-Fat milk and Fresh Berries or Melon on the side)
- Egg Substitute or Egg White Omelet
- Oatmeal (add Nonfat or Low-Fat Milk or nuts for extra protein and Brown sugar for flavor)
- Eggs (their protein content helps keep blood sugars stable, but go easy due to their high cholesterol content and beware of the company they keep)

WITH CAUTION OR RARELY

- Bacon, Ham, Sausage, Hash Browns, Fried Potatoes
- French Toast, Waffles, Pancakes, Eggs Benedict

Salads

YES

- Caesar or Chopped Salad (ask for meat, cheese, and avocado to be limited to 1 ounce and low-fat dressing or dressing on the side; add mild vinegar or lemon juice for additional moisture)
- Spinach Salad (restrictions as above, no bacon)

WITH CAUTION OR RARELY

- Cobb Salad with Full-Fat Dressing and Croutons (ask for meat, cheese, and avocado to be limited to 1 ounce and low-fat dressing or dressing on the side; add mild vinegar or lemon juice for additional moisture)

Soups

YES

- Bean, Lentil, Vegetable, Minestrone, Won Ton, Chicken Noodle (consider a cup rather than a bowl if you want a sandwich or bread with it)
- Black Bean Soup (limit or no sour cream)
- Chili (no cheese)
- Manhattan Clam Chowder (tomato-based)

MAYBE

- Onion Soup (without cheese, or limit cheese to ½ ounce)
- Bread or Crackers (if your calorie count for the day is expected to be low)

BETTER TO SKIP

- Cream Soups
- New England Clam Chowder (cream-based)

Breads

One ounce of bread equals 15 grams of carbohydrates and almost 100 calories; most bread is 1 or 2 ounces per slice, but the range can vary widely. Choose bread only if it fits into your rough expected calorie count for the day.

YES

- Whole-Wheat, Pumpernickel, Rye, Whole-Grain Bread (1 small slice)

WITH CAUTION OR RARELY

- Large Pretzel, Muffin (often 5 ounces or equal to 5 slices of bread; fat-free or not, they're big on calories)

Sandwiches

YES

- Half a Sandwich (ask for bread sliced thin; take the rest home)
- Sliced Turkey, Chicken, Lean Ham or Lean Beef with Lettuce, Tomato, and Mustard (hold the mayonnaise and cheese, and remember, the amount of meat between the bread is as important as the choice of meat)

- Tuna or Chicken Salad (only if little or no mayonnaise is used; always ask for lettuce and tomato)

BETTER TO SKIP

- Full-Sized Deli Sandwich (can represent as many as 8 portions, or 650 calories!)

Mexican Restaurant

YES

- Fajitas (skip the rice and beans, and limit tortillas to 1 or 2)
- Salsa, Chopped Tomato, Shredded Lettuce
- Whole Roasted Fish with Lime
- Chicken or Fish Tacos, not breaded
- Ceviche (marinated raw fish salad)

MAYBE

- Rice or Beans or Tortillas (only if calorie count for the day is low; avoid excessive cheese; don't eat some of each)
- Sour Cream, Guacamole, Cheese (only in tiny amounts, for flavor)

BETTER TO SKIP

- Combo Plates (loaded with starch, calories, cheese, and oil)
- More than 10 Tortilla Chips (ask the server to remove them after 8, for safety)

Italian Restaurant

YES

- Pasta (in small quantities only, i.e., half- or appetizer-sized portion)
- Tomato-Based Sauces (with fish, shellfish, and/or vegetables, if desired)
- Salad (Italian dressing on the side and limit to 1 tablespoon or so)
- Veal Piccata
- Chicken Cacciatore (tomato sauce, without skin by request or do it yourself)
- Grilled Vegetables
- Fish Soup

- Pizza (lean meat, chicken, or vegetarian with very light cheese topping, only if you can afford the calories of 300 to 500 per slice)

- Cream Sauces
- Veal or Chicken Parmigiana

Chinese Restaurant

Hooray for vegetables (fiber, vitamins, minerals, and flavor)!

- Shrimp or Chicken with Snow Peas
- Moo Goo Gai Pan (chicken with vegetables)
- Stir-Fried Vegetables

- Beef with Broccoli (request more broccoli than beef and minimal oil)
- Rice (if you can afford the calories); Fried Rice with minimal oil as an entrée rather than a side
- Pork Dishes (only if lean cuts are used, ask the server)

- Oil-Blanched Meat (such as sweet and sour pork; ask the server if they follow this practice, which makes food very fat-heavy)
- Ordering One Entrée by Yourself (split one with a friend instead)
- Second Helpings

Chicken Restaurant

- Roasted Skinless White Meat
- Vegetable Side Dishes (broccoli, spinach, green beans, carrots)
- Corn or Squash Side Dishes (if you can afford the calories)

- Roasted Skinless Dark Meat (slightly higher in calories and fat grams)

- Fried Chicken
- Roasted Skin-On Chicken
- Creamy Potato Sides
- Creamed Spinach

Fish Restaurant

Watch our for portion size! The Chart House, a popular national restaurant chain that specializes in fresh seafood and steak, says: "Our average dinner portion of fish is eight to nine ounces."

YES
- Shrimp Cocktail
- Steamed Clams or Mussels
- Salmon or any White Fish (grilled, with lemon)

MAYBE
- Shrimp Entrée (if you can afford the cholesterol)

BETTER TO SKIP
- Large Portions (take the other half home)
- Breaded and Fried Fish
- Cream or Butter Sauces

Steak Restaurant

Once thought to be the dieter's choice! Steak surely isn't anymore.

YES
- Flank Steak, Skirt Steak, London Broil (grilled with lemon or salsa, as part of a balanced meal plan)

MAYBE
- New York Strip or Sirloin Steak (grilled as per above)

BETTER TO SKIP
- Prime Rib, Filet Mignon
- Cream Sauces

A Few Surprises

Here is a list of typical restaurant selections with their nutritional values—the numbers may surprise you.

RESTAURANT DISH	CALORIES	FAT	CARBOHYDRATE
Hamburger and Onion Rings	1,550	101	126
Lasagna	960	53	93
Caesar Salad	660	46	30
Porterhouse Steak Dinner (with baked potato, butter, vegetables, salad)	1,860	125	69
Fettuccine Alfredo	1,200	80	98
Mixed Salad with Roquefort Dressing	600	36	45
Club Sandwich	1,222	65	85
Risotto	1,280	110	60

SURVIVING FAST FOOD RESTAURANTS

In light of everyone's busy lives these days, an overview of the best fast food options is in order. The details may be especially beneficial for teens who consider trips to McDonald's, Burger King, and Taco Bell a way of life. A "kid's meal" portion is usually the right amount for both teens and adults—a 2- to 3-ounce hamburger, small fries, and nonfat or low-fat milk or a yogurt cone for roughly 600 calories. A side salad is a nice addition. Another quick acceptable meal is a grilled chicken sandwich (not breaded) with lots of tomato, lettuce, and onions, a little barbecue sauce or ketchup, and nonfat or low-fat milk. A simple hamburger, taco, or sandwich plus a diet drink or iced tea should also keep your calories down to between 300 and 500.

Remember that a quarter-pound hamburger or cheeseburger with one bun can be more filling and lower in calories than anything in a triple-decker bun. But hold off on that breaded fish sandwich—it's not a better choice than a hamburger (a popular misconception). Breading acts as a grease sponge, and as a rule of thumb, doubles the food's calorie value. Here's how the two sandwiches compare:

SANDWICH	CALORIES	FAT	CARBOHYDRATE
McDonald's Fish Sandwich	440	26	38
McDonald's Plain Hamburger	260	10	31

Don't assume a trip through the salad bar will net you less fat and fewer calories than ordering a sandwich. It all depends on what you choose. Most of these quick-service establishments are sorely lacking fresh fruits and vegetables, so make up for them at other meals throughout the day. Low-fat milk provides the same amount of calcium as a thick shake, but with two-thirds fewer calories (only 130 calories in an 8-ounce carton). Or order a frozen yogurt cone at 120 calories rather than a 16-ounce shake at McDonald's for 300 to 500 calories. Finally, do try to avoid fries, or at least stick with the smallest order. Better yet, share an order with a friend.

This may seem like a lot of information to absorb, but reading through this chapter you'll see that making sensible restaurant choices is mostly just common sense. When dining out, you're the boss. Order half portions, grilled fish, or whatever you need to make your lunch or dinner a healthy option within your personal meal plan. If the restaurant is less than obliging, choose another, nicer establishment. Stick to the basics: If you avoid ordering complicated or saucy dishes, you'll be able to see exactly what's on the plate and thus assess the calories.

Whether you go to a sit-down restaurant or a fast food drive-through, remember that portion control is everything. Don't hesitate to wrap up half your meal if you are exceeding the recommended portion—or leave it on the table.

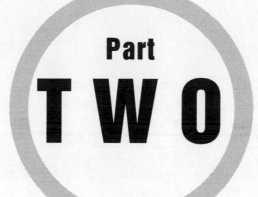

Part
TWO

CHAPTER 10
A New Way
of Cooking

As an ex-smoker on the road to good health, there is no better way to nurture yourself than to prepare a delicious, wholesome meal at home. Haven't been cooking much lately? Feel a little overwhelmed by the idea? Rest assured, the recipes that follow present an approach to cooking that will make your life easier, not harder. You won't be spending hours in the kitchen creating elaborate dishes and multiple courses from scratch. Instead, these recipes will show you how to assemble a few fresh, simple ingredients, perhaps with some ready-prepared items, to create gourmet meals in very little time. They'll also help you turn one meal into two or three by using the extras from your weekend cooking as the basis for quick weekday dinners.

MENU PLANNING

People who tend to binge are more likely to resist that temptation if they choose well-balanced meals over a single food such as popcorn, rice cakes, or cereal. To create a balanced meal, you must include adequate amounts of protein, which gives you a greater sense of fullness during the course of a meal than an equal amount of carbohydrate. Include fat, which enhances the sense of fullness between meals. Also, make sure to eat a variety of foods, such as vegetables, salads, fruit, and whole-grain breads, plus lean protein or legumes and nuts. Featuring all the food groups goes a long way toward making you feel satisfied; dietary fiber also helps increase the feeling of fullness. And warm foods are usually more satisfying than cold foods or foods eaten at room temperature. With these guidelines, you can pamper yourself in a smart way rather than with a bowl of caramel popcorn.

THE SHORTCUT KITCHEN

It's a good idea to shop for groceries at least once a week so you always have fresh ingredients available for a quick and appealing meal. In addition, stock up on healthy pantry items that will make impromptu cooking easier. Keeping basic ingredients on hand means you can use these elements to prepare spur-of-the-moment meals. Many staple ingredients are flavorful, versatile, and easy to use. Follow the recipes in this book, or simply use them as a starting point. Let your creativity take over and you'll soon learn to combine ingredients in a variety of ways to come up with a fabulous selection of healthy meals. The items listed below are all excellent bets; keep a good assortment in your kitchen at all times.

Meat, Poultry, and Fish

Select lean cuts of beef, pork, ham, and the like, with minimal fat marbling. Unless you're planning to freeze them, buy only what you will need until the next shopping trip; be sure to note the sell-by date. Freeze meat, fish, and chicken in individual or family-sized packets to keep on hand for longer periods.

Delicatessen Meats

Buy sliced meats such as oven-roasted turkey and chicken breast, lean ham, or roast beef.

Fresh Fruit

Again, limit your supply to the amount to be used in the near future. Apples, pears, oranges, not-too-ripe bananas, melons, plums, and nectarines are ideal. Lemons and limes add a welcome zing and last longer than other fruits.

Fresh Vegetables

Great choices include broccoli, cauliflower, eggplant, mushrooms, sugar snap peas, zucchini, celery, carrots, cabbage, tomatoes, and salad greens. Less perishable produce like potatoes, winter squash, onions, and garlic can be kept at room temperature.

Grain, Cereals, and Breads

Pasta (fresh or dried); rice (white, brown, minute rice); couscous; quick-cooking or old-fashioned oats; shredded wheat and other low-fat, high-fiber cereals; whole-wheat bread; pita bread; English muffins.

Refrigerator Staples

Ready-made pizza crusts (can also be bought frozen); reduced-fat flour and corn tortillas; jarred roasted red peppers and pimientos; low-fat cheese (Cheddar, Parmesan, mozzarella); yogurt (nonfat plain or flavored); pickled ginger (sushi style); eggs; 1% fat cottage cheese; buttermilk; Dijon mustard; peanut butter; capers.

Frozen Foods

Vegetables such as corn, peas, green beans, and spinach; fruits like strawberries, blueberries, and raspberries; snacks like juice bars, sorbet, frozen yogurt, and low-fat ice cream.

Ready-Made Sauces and Flavor-Boosting Condiments

Pasta sauces like marinara or pesto (refrigerated or bottled); ethnic sauces and flavoring pastes like soy sauce, hoisin sauce, plum sauce, curry paste, olive paste, fish sauce, and bottled salsa; seasoned rice wine vinegar, balsamic vinegar, and flavored vinegars like champagne and raspberry; Marsala wine, sherry, vermouth, white and/or red wine; Tabasco or other hot pepper sauce; black and green olives; jalapeño peppers.

The Pantry

Canned tomato paste, tomato puree, tomato sauce, and whole tomatoes; canned low-fat, low-sodium chicken, beef, and vegetable broth; canned beans (garbanzo, kidney, black, white); canned water-packed tuna, canned jalapeño and mild green chili peppers; wheat germ; bread crumbs; corn bread mix; powdered soup mixes; chocolate chips; raisins or currants; dried fruit.

MAINTAINING THE SHORTCUT KITCHEN

Using the suggestions above as a guide, make your own "stand-by" shopping list. Replenish the pantry, refrigerator, and freezer as you use up ingredients; keep a running list of items that are getting low so you can remember to buy them the next time you shop. Organization is the key to simple and successful meal preparation.

HEALTHY QUICK-FIX MEAL IDEAS

- Thin pasta such as dried spaghettini cooks quickly and makes a delicious main dish with leftover cooked vegetables and lean meat. Or use fresh pasta, which cooks even faster, and toss with thawed frozen peas, chopped canned tomatoes, and a handful of capers. Or, top cooked pasta with ready-made pasta sauce such as pesto or marinara, a few shavings of fresh Parmesan cheese, and lots of black pepper.
- Cook rice in low-fat, low-sodium chicken broth instead of water, with a bit of minced garlic for extra flavor. Stir in lean cooked (or leftover) meat, diced cooked vegetables, or drained canned beans.
- Used canned beans, such as pintos or black beans to fill quesadillas or burritos. They provide welcome texture and good nutrition, too. Add some sprouts or shredded lettuce, a little low-fat cheese, and a dollop of salsa.
- To add quick taste, texture and crunch, toss honey-coated wheat germ or a few chopped peanuts or walnuts into 1% fat cottage cheese, low-fat yogurt, and fruit salads.
- Flavor fish, chicken, or pork chops with bottled sauces like salsa, pesto, or chutney for instant gourmet taste.
- Use packaged and cut fresh vegetables, prepared salad greens, and ready-made cabbage slaws for fast side dishes and stir-fries. Add strips of ham or deli-roast chicken for a full meal. Seasoned rice wine vinegar makes a great topping.

- Add frozen spinach, corn, or peas to soups or cooked pasta or fry them with leftover rice for quick fried rice. Remember to keep oil to 1 teaspoon per person.
- Add salsa, grated low-fat cheese, and mushrooms to beaten egg whites or liquid egg substitute for a quick and tasty omelet.
- Wrap leftover fish, chicken, meat, and/or beans in a reduced-fat tortilla to make a satisfying burrito or "wrap." Heat in a microwave, if desired.

SIMPLE SECRETS TO SHORTCUT COOKING

Once your pantry, refrigerator, and freezer are stocked and organized, assembling quick meals in a hurry is a cinch. Just apply some basic principles and use a few timesaving tips.

- Make two meals out of one by preparing extra pancakes, French toast, muffins, or even oatmeal (try the Baked Oatmeal on page 153) — reheat leftovers for the next day's breakfast.
- Prepare sandwich fillings such as tuna or chicken salad in larger quantities to provide two or three lunches.
- Whenever you make a salad, clean all the greens, the entire head of broccoli, the whole bag of carrots, and so on, even if you don't intend to use them all immediately. Just store in Ziploc bags or plastic containers in the crisper section of your refrigerator, and the next salad (or stir-fry or vegetable side dish) will be much easier.
- When you need just half a bell pepper or onion, trim and chop the whole vegetable, refrigerate the extra in a plastic bag, and use within a day or two.
- Steam more vegetables than you plan to eat and use the extras as cold snacks or in salads. You can also puree them in a blender or food processor with some low-fat milk, buttermilk, or broth for a quick soup. This soup idea works well with broccoli (see page 173), cauliflower, and corn.

- Make soups from scratch (see page 181) in a double or triple batch—they're a great way to use up leftover vegetables as well as pasta. Freeze the amount you don't intend to eat within the next several days.
- Prepare extra boneless, skinless chicken breasts for sandwiches, lunches, or tortilla wraps. Sliced or cubed cooked chicken is also good tossed into pasta sauces, rice dishes, or salads.
- Eat a hamburger at home—it's a great way to satisfy a red-meat craving without all the fat of a restaurant burger. Cook extra burgers (lean beef or turkey), and then reheat in the microwave for another meal.
- Use extra cooked, flaked fish in sandwiches, salads, or tortillas.
- Cook extra pasta, without a sauce, and reheat it for another meal. Store plain cooked pasta in a Ziploc bag. To heat and separate, rinse it in a sieve or colander with boiling water.
- Cook extra rice, cover, and refrigerate. The next day, transform it into fried rice with the addition of a few vegetables and perhaps a beaten egg (see page 252).
- Steam or bake double the amount of potatoes you plan to eat for another potato dish later in the week. Try them mashed or made into potato pancakes (see page 254).

You'll be amazed at the versatility of a well-stocked pantry—and the delicious "shortcut" dishes you can create using these tips. Following are 100 quick and easy recipes for every meal, including breakfasts, lunches, weeknight suppers and more elaborate weekend dinners, plus several "instant" weekday recipes that use convenience ingredients and extra-easy cooking techniques.

CHAPTER 11
Breakfast
and Brunch

If you're like most people, your mom told you that breakfast is the most important meal of the day. Well, guess what? She was right. If you've been in the habit of having coffee and a cigarette instead of a real breakfast, learning the advantages to the latter may motivate a change in your morning routine.

WHY DO I HAVE TO EAT BREAKFAST?

First, people who skip breakfast are likely to have more body fat, gain more weight (or lose less), and have higher blood cholesterol levels than those who eat breakfast. Also, the right combination of foods in the morning helps stabilize your blood sugar, making you less likely to overeat later in the day. If you just can't face food in the morning, try redefining breakfast as something to eat sometime midmorning rather than the moment you wake up.

WHAT MAKES A GOOD BREAKFAST?

Breakfast should include carbohydrates and protein for stabilizing the blood sugar levels and stopping you from getting hungry again too quickly. Baked Oatmeal (page 153) made with milk, an egg white omelet (page 158) served with whole-grain toast, or Ranch-Style Eggs with Tortillas (page 162) are ideal carbohydrate-protein combinations. Smoothies feature yogurt or buttermilk as the high-protein base, with fruit as a carbohydrate boost. Have a glass of nonfat or low-fat milk or make your coffee into a latte for extra protein, then add a Honey-Bran Blueberry Muffin (page 154) or a slice of Peanut Butter-Banana Toast (page 160). You'll have no trouble eating breakfast with these delicious goodies to choose from.

Note that any ingredients listed as optional have not been included in the nutritional calculation. Today's nutritional labeling makes it simple to add the calories from, for instance, a spoonful of sugar-free maple syrup or a dollop of low-fat sour cream.

BAKED OATMEAL

SERVES 4

*I*f you like bread pudding, you'll love this version made with oats instead of bread. Enjoy it with low-calorie, sugar-free maple syrup. For oatmeal fans who don't want to take the time to make oatmeal during the week, make a double batch of this tasty dish on the weekend, then simply heat for your breakfast during the week.

1 cup quick-cooking oats or 1½ cups old-fashioned oats

½ cup (firmly packed) light or dark brown sugar

½ teaspoon ground cinnamon

½ teaspoon salt (optional)

2 large egg whites or ¼ cup liquid egg substitute

1½ cups nonfat milk

1 tablespoon vegetable oil

1 teaspoon vanilla extract

Sugar-free maple syrup or nonfat yogurt for serving (optional)

1. Preheat the oven to 350°F. Spray an 8 × 4-inch loaf pan with vegetable oil.
2. In a large bowl, mix together the oats, brown sugar, cinnamon, and salt.
3. In a medium bowl, whisk together the egg whites, milk, oil, and vanilla. Add the milk mixture to the flour mixture and stir until well blended.
4. Pour the mixture into the prepared baking pan. Bake for 40 to 45 minutes, until the center is set and firm to the touch. Cool slightly before serving with sugar-free syrup or yogurt, if desired. Store, covered, in the refrigerator for up to 3 days.

Per Serving: calories, 225; fat (g), 5; carbohydrates (g), 37; protein (g), 8; cholesterol (mg), 2; sodium (mg), 350.

HEALTH CHECK
• High in fiber, oats will keep you feeling full longer than other foods with a similar calorie content.
• The protein in milk and egg whites will help keep blood sugars stable well into the morning, and thus keep hunger in check at lunchtime.
• The fiber in oats helps lower blood cholesterol levels, which are often elevated in smokers and new ex-smokers.

PEANUT BUTTER-
BANANA TOAST

SERVES 4

*T*he combination of peanut butter and banana is a "natural," and one
that's delicious. Add a sugar and cinnamon topping, toast it all, and you have
an extra-special treat. Be sure to use a good-quality whole-grain bread that
will keep its form.

4 slices whole-grain bread	**1 teaspoon sugar**
2 tablespoons peanut butter	**⅛ teaspoon ground cinnamon**
2 ripe bananas	

1. Preheat a broiler or toaster oven. Toast the bread until golden, then cool
briefly. Spread each slice of toast with 1½ teaspoons of peanut butter.
2. Halve each banana crosswise. Slice each half lengthwise into 2 or 3 pieces.
Lay the banana slices on the toast, overlapping them if necessary.
3. Mix together the sugar and cinnamon and sprinkle about ¼ teaspoon of
the mixture evenly over each piece of banana toast.
4. Place on a pan and toast under the broiler or in the toaster oven for 1 to 2
minutes, until the sugar has melted and the tops are lightly browned. Watch
closely, as they can scorch quickly. Cool briefly, then cut each slice of toast in
half on the diagonal. Serve warm.

Per Serving (1 slice): calories, 185; fat (g), 6; carbohydrates (g), 31; protein (g), 6;
cholesterol (mg), 0; sodium (mg), 170.

HEALTH CHECK

• Whole grains give a boost of fiber with relatively few calories—they're a great
alternative when you're tempted to reach for a cigarette.
• Bananas are a good source of vitamin B_6, which is often compromised in
smokers' diets.
• Recent studies show that the chemical galanin, which is present in the appetite
control center of the brain, may be responsible for our fat cravings. Created when
you eat fat, galanin makes you crave fats even more. Eating just a little fat can help
satisfy the urge. This breakfast has just enough fat to appease a craving without a
calorie overload.

BUTTERMILK PANCAKES

MAKES 8 TO 9 PANCAKES; SERVES 2

*W*eekends call for a little change of pace. Make the time to sit down to a splurge of pancakes instead of the usual on-the-go bagels or toast. These pancakes are deliciously light and fluffy, with a savory hint of cinnamon and buttermilk, but they're low in fat, so no "guilties."

1¼ cups low-fat buttermilk	½ teaspoon baking soda
1 large egg	¼ teaspoon ground cinnamon
1 cup all-purpose flour	¼ teaspoon salt
1 tablespoon sugar	Warm sugar-free maple syrup
¾ teaspoon baking powder	for serving (optional)

1. Preheat the oven to 200°F. In a medium bowl, combine the buttermilk and egg until well mixed.
2. In a separate bowl, mix together the flour, sugar, baking powder, baking soda, cinnamon, and salt. Add the buttermilk mixture to the flour mixture and stir until just combined. Be sure not to overmix or the pancakes will be tough.
3. Spray a griddle or large nonstick skillet with vegetable oil spray, then heat over medium heat. Ladle about ¼ cup of batter per pancake onto the griddle or skillet. Spread the batter with the back of a spoon to thin slightly.
4. Cook, for 2 to 3 minutes, until a few bubbles break on the top. Turn and cook for about 2 minutes more, until browned on the underside. Transfer to an ovenproof plate and keep warm in the oven while cooking the remaining pancakes. Serve hot, with warm maple syrup, if desired.

Per Serving (4 pancakes; without syrup): calories, 350; fat (g), 5; carbohydrates (g), 62; protein (g), 15; cholesterol (mg), 112; sodium (mg), 960.

HEALTH CHECK
• Look for reduced-calorie maple syrups, which are as much as 70 percent lower in calories.
• Starting your day with a high-carbohydrate food such as pancakes will boost your body's level of serotonin, which calms you down and may decrease your craving for a cigarette.
• Distinctively tangy low-fat buttermilk replaces whole milk and saves calories.

CRANBERRY-OATMEAL MUFFINS

MAKES 12 MUFFINS

*T*hese muffins combine the tart taste of cranberries with the heartiness of oats—a terrific combination. Dried blueberries or cherries can be substituted for the cranberries, if you prefer.

1 cup all-purpose flour	1 cup old-fashioned oats
1 cup sugar	2 large egg whites
1 tablespoon baking powder	1 cup low-fat buttermilk
½ teaspoon baking soda	¼ cup canola oil
Pinch of salt	1 cup dried cranberries

1. Position the rack in the center of the oven and preheat to 375°F. Spray a 12-cup nonstick muffin pan with vegetable oil spray.

2. In a large bowl, sift together the flour, sugar, baking powder, baking soda, and salt. Add the oats and mix to combine thoroughly.

3. In another bowl or a large glass measuring jug, whisk together the egg whites, buttermilk and oil until evenly blended.

4. Add the buttermilk mixture to the flour mixture and stir until just combined. Be sure not to overmix, and don't worry if there are a few lumps. Fold the cranberries gently into the batter with a large rubber spatula.

5. Divide the batter equally among the prepared muffin cups. Bake for about 20 minutes, or until the muffins are golden and a toothpick inserted into the center of one of them comes out clean. Transfer the pan to a wire rack and cool for at least 10 minutes before removing the muffins. Serve warm or at room temperature.

Per Serving (1 muffin): calories, 180; fat (g), 5; carbohydrates (g), 30; protein (g), 3; cholesterol (mg), 0; sodium (mg), 230.

HEALTH CHECK

• High in fiber, oats will keep you feeling full longer than other foods with a similar calorie content.

• The fiber in oats may help lower cholesterol levels in the blood. This is an important bonus for smokers, who are at a greater risk for heart disease.

• People who have recently stopped smoking may have more insulin circulating in their blood, which may increase the craving for sweets. A small quantity of sugar in a low-fat food can help without a calorie overload.

CRUNCHY GRANOLA

SERVES 4

*M*any commercial granolas are high in fat—just read the labels. This one, however, contains little fat and is very tasty, so making your own is definitely worthwhile. Keep a stash of this crunchy granola in your office for snacks. It's also good for breakfast topped with milk and sliced fresh fruit.

½ cup honey

¼ cup water

1 tablespoon canola oil

½ teaspoon vanilla extract

1½ cups high-fiber, low-fat
   ready-to-eat cereal

1 cup quick-cooking or old-
   fashioned oats

½ cup powdered nonfat milk

¼ teaspoon ground cinnamon

¼ teaspoon salt (optional)

1. Preheat the oven to 350°F. Cover a 15 × 10-inch jelly-roll pan or rimmed baking sheet with aluminum foil and spray lightly with vegetable oil spray.
2. In a small saucepan, combine the honey, water, oil, and vanilla, then stir over low heat until the honey is melted. In a large bowl, combine the cereal, oats, powdered milk, cinnamon, and, if desired, the salt.
3. Drizzle the honey mixture over the cereal mixture, stirring until evenly coated. Spread the mixture evenly in the prepared jelly-roll pan.
4. Bake for 10 minutes, then stir. Bake for 10 minutes more, or until golden brown. Transfer the pan to a wire rack and cool the granola completely. Store, tightly covered, at room temperature for up to 1 week.

Per Serving (1 cup): calories, 270; fat (g), 5; carbohydrates (g), 55; protein (g), 7; cholesterol (mg), 2; sodium (mg), 280.

HEALTH CHECK
- Granola provides a satisfying crunch that helps soothe the need for oral gratification.
- The fiber in oats may help lower cholesterol levels in the blood. Smokers, who are at a greater risk for heart disease, will especially benefit from this.
- Vanilla extract is a versatile ingredient that adds tons of flavor without fat or calories.

EGG WHITE OMELET WITH GREEN ONION AND PARMESAN

SERVES 1

*Y*ou'll be surprised at how little you miss the yolk when a few seasonings are added to this delicious egg-white-only omelet. Buy large or jumbo eggs to obtain the maximum egg white per egg. For other recipes that call for whole eggs, buy small or medium eggs, which could technically be marketed as "low-cholesterol." Take the liberty of adding any leftover cooked vegetables that you have on hand, such as spinach, carrots, or zucchini.

4 large or jumbo egg whites

1 tablespoon grated Parmesan
   cheese

1 green onion (scallion), white

and light green parts only,
   thinly sliced

Salt and black pepper to taste

1. In a small bowl, beat the egg whites until frothy. Stir in the cheese and set aside. Spray a medium nonstick skillet with vegetable oil spray and heat over medium-high heat. Add the green onion and cook for about 2 minutes, or until slightly softened.

2. Pour in the egg white mixture. Rotate the pan to coat the bottom evenly with the egg whites, pulling back the cooked edges of the omelet to let the uncooked portion flow underneath.

3. Continue cooking for about 2 minutes, or until the top is set. Fold the omelet in half, using a fork or nonstick spatula to ease one side over the other. Season with salt and pepper and serve immediately.

Per Serving: calories, 97; fat (g), 2; carbohydrates (g), 2; protein (g), 17; cholesterol (mg), 5; sodium (mg), 340.

HEALTH CHECK

• The protein in egg whites will help keep blood sugars stable well into the morning, and thus keep hunger in check at lunchtime.

• At less than 100 calories per serving, this is a good option for those trying to avoid weight gain.

• Substituting egg whites for yolks means less cholesterol in the diet, an important goal for smokers because of their greater risk of heart disease.

FRENCH TOAST

SERVES 4

*A*ny type of bread works well with this recipe, particularly if it's a day or two old and has begun to dry out. Experiment with raisin bread or your favorite whole-grain variety.

1 large egg
2 large egg whites
¼ cup nonfat milk
½ teaspoon vanilla extract
Pinch of ground cinnamon
8 1-inch-thick, diagonally cut

slices of French, Italian, or whole-grain bread
½ cup sugar-free maple syrup, for serving (2 tablespoons per serving)

1. Preheat the oven to 200°F. In a shallow dish, beat the whole egg and egg whites with a wire whisk or fork until foamy. Add the milk, vanilla, and cinnamon. Blend thoroughly and set aside.
2. Lightly spray a large nonstick skillet with vegetable oil spray and heat over medium heat. Dip 4 of the bread slices into the egg mixture, turning to coat them well. Drain the excess egg mixture back into the dish.
3. Place the dipped slices in the skillet and cook for about 2 minutes per side, or until golden brown, turning once.
4. Transfer to an ovenproof plate and keep warm in the oven. Dip the remaining slices in the egg mixture and cook as above. Spray the skillet with more vegetable oil spray as needed. Top the French toast with maple syrup and serve hot.

Per Serving (2 slices): calories, 275; fat (g), 3; carbohydrates (g), 54; protein (g), 8; cholesterol (mg), 54; sodium (mg), 360.

HEALTH CHECK
• Starting your day with a high-carbohydrate food such as French toast with syrup will boost your body's level of serotonin, which calms you down and may decrease your craving for a cigarette.
• The protein in egg whites will help keep blood sugars stable well into the morning, and thus keep hunger in check at lunchtime.
• Replacing whole milk with nonfat milk reduces fat, which prevents weight gain and cuts the risk of heart disease, a concern for smokers.

HONEY-BRAN BLUEBERRY MUFFINS

MAKES 12 MUFFINS

*T*hese delicious muffins are a filling breakfast or snack. Add a slice of low-fat cheddar cheese and a glass of nonfat milk for a sense of fullness.

1 cup all-purpose flour

1 cup unprocessed wheat bran

1 tablespoon baking powder

¾ teaspoon salt

½ teaspoon baking soda

2 large egg whites

1 cup low-fat buttermilk

¼ cup honey

2 tablespoons canola oil

¼ teaspoon vanilla extract

1 cup fresh or thawed frozen
  blueberries

1. Position a rack in the center of the oven and preheat to 400°F. Line a 12-cup muffin pan with paper muffin liners or spray the cups with vegetable oil spray.

2. In a large bowl, mix together the flour, wheat bran, baking powder, salt, and baking soda. In a medium bowl, whisk together the egg whites, buttermilk, honey, oil, and vanilla.

3. Add the buttermilk mixture to the flour mixture and stir until just combined. Be sure not to overmix, and don't worry if a few lumps remain. Fold the blueberries gently into the batter with a large rubber spatula.

4. Divide the batter equally among the prepared muffin cups. Bake for about 20 minutes, or until the muffins are golden brown and a toothpick inserted into the center of one of them comes out clean. Transfer the pan to a wire rack and cool for at least 15 minutes. Serve warm or at room temperature.

Per Serving (1 muffin): calories, 100; fat (g), 3; carbohydrates (g), 18; protein (g), 3; cholesterol (mg), 0; sodium (mg), 340.

HEALTH CHECK

• With only 3 grams of fat per muffin, these are a low-fat option, important for smokers because of cholesterol concerns.

• Wheat bran gives a boost of the kind of fiber that helps keep you regular, always a good thing whether you're a smoker or not. Fiber also increases a sense of fullness.

• Deliciously tangy, low-fat buttermilk replaces whole milk and some of the oil, saving calories and fat grams.

ORANGE-BANANA BREAKFAST SMOOTHIE

SERVES 1

*T*his is the breakfast I choose when dinner the night before was a heavy hitter on carbohydrates like pasta. The variations are endless, particularly if you keep bags of frozen fruit such as strawberries, blueberries, or mangoes in your freezer.

1 orange, cut into pieces and
   seeded if necessary
1 banana, cut into chunks
½ cup nonfat milk or yogurt

4 ice cubes
2 tablespoons honey-toasted
   wheat germ (optional)

In a blender, combine the orange, banana, milk, ice cubes, and, if desired, the wheat germ. Blend until smooth and frothy, pour into a glass, and serve.

Per Serving: calories, 265; fat (g), 2.5; carbohydrates (g), 55; protein (g), 11; cholesterol (mg), 2; sodium (mg), 70.

HEALTH CHECK
• Replacing whole milk with nonfat milk or yogurt reduces fat, which prevents weight gain and cuts the risk of heart disease, an important concern for smokers.
• Fruit gives a boost of fiber with relatively few calories—it's a great alternative when you're tempted to reach for a cigarette.
• Orange adds a shot of vitamin C, which is usually lacking in smokers' diets.

RANCH-STYLE EGGS WITH TORTILLAS

*W*hat a wonderful way to clean out your vegetable bin! You can scramble almost any vegetable into this festive breakfast or brunch dish. For a truly hearty start to your day, serve it with a side of lean ham. The nutritional values on the facing page are based on using an egg substitute; if you use whole large eggs, each serving will contain 300 calories, 216 milligrams of cholesterol, and an additional 3 grams of fat.

6 medium reduced-fat flour tortillas

1 tablespoon olive oil

1 large russet potato (about 13 ounces), baked, peeled, and thinly sliced

1 medium onion, thinly sliced

1 medium zucchini, thinly sliced

½ medium red bell pepper, seeded and diced

1½ cups liquid egg substitute or 6 large eggs

¼ cup nonfat milk

Salt and pepper to taste

¼ cup grated Parmesan cheese

1 tablespoon chopped fresh parsley (optional)

1. Preheat the oven to 200°F. Wrap the tortillas in aluminum foil and place in the oven to warm through.

2. Heat the oil in a large nonstick skillet over medium-high heat. Add the potato, onion, zucchini, and bell pepper and cook for 3 to 4 minutes, until softened.

3. While the vegetables are cooking, in a medium bowl, whisk together the egg substitute, milk, salt, and pepper. Reduce the heat to medium-low and pour the egg mixture over the cooked vegetables. Sprinkle with the cheese and cook, turning and scrambling occasionally, for about 5 minutes, or until the eggs are just set and golden. Do not overcook.

4. Slide the eggs and vegetables onto a platter and sprinkle with the parsley, if desired. Serve with the warm tortillas.

Per Serving: calories, 280; fat (g), 8; carbohydrates (g), 37; protein (g), 15; cholesterol (mg), 4; sodium (mg), 370.

HEALTH CHECK
• Bell peppers and potatoes are both good sources of vitamin C, which is usually low in the blood of smokers.
• Fresh vegetables give a boost of fiber with relatively few calories, a great alternative when you're tempted to reach for a cigarette.
• Starting your day with a high-carbohydrate food such as tortillas will boost your body's level of serotonin, which calms you down and may decrease your craving for a cigarette.
• Eggs add protein, which helps keep blood sugar levels stable and hunger in check.

REFRIGERATOR BUTTERMILK BRAN MUFFINS

MAKES 48 MUFFINS

*T*his recipe has stood the test of time, literally. My mother made these muffins when I was a little girl, and today she makes them for her grandchildren. The uncooked mixture keeps in the refrigerator for up to six weeks, so you can pop a dozen muffins in the oven on the spur of the moment for hot, delicious treats.

4 cups All-Bran cereal	1 cup (firmly packed) brown
2 cups boiling water	sugar
4 cups all-purpose flour	1 cup canola oil
3 tablespoons baking soda	4 large eggs
2 teaspoons salt	1 quart low-fat buttermilk
1¾ cups granulated sugar	2 cups Grape-Nuts cereal

1. Preheat the oven to 400°F. Spray a 12-cup muffin pan with vegetable oil spray or line the muffin cups with paper muffin liners. In a large bowl, combine the All-Bran cereal and boiling water and set aside.

2. In a large plastic storage container, mix together the flour, baking soda, and salt.

3. In a separate bowl, whisk thoroughly together the granulated sugar, brown sugar, oil, and eggs. Add the buttermilk and stir to mix. Add the buttermilk mixture to the flour mixture and stir until just combined. Be sure not to overmix.

4. Add the soaked All-Bran and Grape-Nuts and stir just until combined. Bake the muffins right away, or cover and refrigerate the batter for up to 6 weeks.

5. Spoon the batter into the prepared muffin cups, filling them one-third full and using about ¼ cup of batter for each muffin. Bake for about 20 minutes, or until the muffins are golden brown and a toothpick inserted into the

center of one of them comes out clean. Transfer the pan to a wire rack and cool. Repeat with the remaining batter until all is used, if desired.

Per Serving (1 muffin): calories, 165; fat (g), 5; carbohydrates (g), 28; protein (g), 4; cholesterol (mg), 19; sodium (mg), 420.

HEALTH CHECK

• The protein in buttermilk and eggs will help keep blood sugars stable well into the morning, and thus keep hunger in check at lunchtime.

• This recipe uses canola oil, which has the least amount of saturated fat of all oils and no cholesterol, a bonus for smokers because of their increased risk for heart disease.

• Only 5 grams of fat per muffin is a good value for those trying to avoid weight gain.

CHAPTER 12
Appetizers

Smoking occupies your hands. You know the routine: extracting a cigarette, perhaps tapping it on a counter, and then lighting it. This is a pattern that you were very familiar with, perhaps for a long time. When you stop performing that routine, you may feel a sense of loss and not know what to do with your hands. You are also accustomed to putting things in your mouth. Add it all up and it's clear why many who quit smoking tend to snack a lot. It's an activity that involves the hands, the mouth, and the pleasure centers of the brain—i.e., just like smoking. But because most snack foods are high in calories and fat, satisfying those needs is likely to cause weight gain. Fortunately, there are ways to meet your needs for oral stimulation and hand-to-mouth activity without gaining weight, and here are some tasty appetizers to get you started. In the snacking chapter (pages 116–129), there are many more ideas for "safe snacking" that don't require a recipe.

If you serve appetizers before a meal, be sure to compensate by eating less food when dinner comes around. To accompany cocktails—which could be a time when you're tempted to smoke—reach instead for a portion of Ham with Melon (page 168) or Vegetable Dip for Crudités (page 170).

ARTICHOKES WITH DIP
SERVES 2

*E*ating an artichoke—plucking off each leaf and dunking them one by one in the dip—is a great activity that results in very few calories and a considerable passage of time. If you've never done it, here's a simple recipe. It's just the reward you deserve for taking on a healthier lifestyle. This recipe suggests steaming the artichokes, but if you don't have a large enough steamer, simply cook them directly in the water.

2 large artichokes (4 ounces each)
¼ cup light mayonnaise

1 tablespoon fresh lemon juice
Salt and black pepper to taste

1. Trim off the tough bottom of each artichoke stem, then pull off the lower, tough outer leaves. Trim off the tips of the artichoke leaves with scissors. In a large pot fitted with a steamer insert, place just enough water to hit the bottom of the steamer. Bring the water to a boil. Place the artichokes in the steamer basket.
2. Cover and simmer for about 30 minutes, or until the artichoke bases are tender when pierced with a knife and the outer leaves pull away easily.
3. While the artichokes are cooking, prepare the dip: In a small bowl, mix together the mayonnaise, lemon, salt, and pepper.
4. When the artichokes are cooked, drain them thoroughly. Place each artichoke on a plate, with some dip on the side, and serve.

Per Serving: calories, 160; fat (g), 10; carbohydrates (g), 16; protein (g), 4; cholesterol (mg), 10; sodium (mg), 480.

HEALTH CHECK
• Fresh artichokes add a boost of fiber with relatively few calories, a great alternative when you're tempted to reach for a cigarette.
• Using light mayonnaise instead of regular reduces the fat in this dish by half without compromising flavor. For an even lighter version, use low-fat instead of light mayonnaise.
• If you're tempted to pick up a cigarette just to have something in your hands and mouth, try this instead.

HAM WITH MELON
SERVES 4

*W*hen you're looking for a low-calorie, filling snack to replace the urge for a cigarette, this is a great one. The saltiness and little bit of fat in the ham, though very satisfying, are no cause for the "guilties." Just keep cantaloupe and lean ham in your refrigerator. Papaya, pineapple, or mango work well, too.

2 thin slices lean ham   **4 small slices cantaloupe**

Halve each ham slice lengthwise, then wrap each half slice around a melon slice. If desired, skewer with a toothpick to hold the ham. Refrigerate for up to 20 minutes before serving.

Per Serving: calories, 15; fat (g), less than 1 g; carbohydrates (g), 1; protein (g), 2; cholesterol (mg), 3; sodium (mg), 100.

HEALTH CHECK
• Each serving has less than 1 gram of fat, but lots of flavor.
• Cantaloupe is high in vitamins A and C, antioxidants that help to destroy the process that can create cancer cells.
• This elegant dish supplies a whole day's worth of several vitamins plus lots of potassium.

REFRIED BEAN DIP

MAKES 2½ CUPS

*S*erve this tasty dip with reduced-fat tortillas or tortilla chips. Butter-milk is a clever way to add a cheeselike flavor without the fat. The result is better than any dip I've ever eaten in a restaurant.

4 green onions (scallions), white and light green parts only, finely chopped

1 16-ounce can fat-free refried pinto or black beans

½ cup low-fat buttermilk

1 4-ounce can chopped mild green chilies, drained

½ teaspoon ground cumin

Dash of hot sauce (optional)

1. Lightly spray a large nonstick skillet with vegetable oil spray and heat over medium heat. Add the green onions and cook for about 1 minute, or until just heated through. Stir in the beans, buttermilk, chilies, and cumin until smooth. Taste for seasoning and add the hot sauce, if desired. Transfer to a serving bowl and let cool.

2. Cover and refrigerate for 2 to 6 hours to allow the flavors to blend. Bring back to room temperature before serving.

Per Serving (¼ cup): calories, 100; fat (g), 0; carbohydrates (g), 20; protein (g), 7; cholesterol (mg), 1; sodium (mg), 630.

HEALTH CHECK

• The protein in beans will help keep blood sugars stable well into the afternoon, and thus keep hunger in check at dinner.

• Beans give a boost of soluble fiber—the kind that helps lower blood cholesterol levels—an important benefit for smokers, who are at a greater risk for heart disease.

• Low-fat buttermilk is a healthy and rich-tasting alternative to cheese or whole milk in this recipe.

VEGETABLE DIP FOR CRUDITÉS

MAKES 4 CUPS

*A*rtichoke dip seems to be showing up in restaurants everywhere, so I decided to do a light version. Canned artichoke hearts make quick work of this recipe, and the spinach adds a little extra color and nutrition. The nutritional analysis is for the dip only—raw vegetables will add a few calories.

1 8-ounce package light cream cheese, at room temperature

1 cup part-skim ricotta cheese

1 cup (packed) thawed, drained frozen spinach

½ cup grated Parmesan cheese

1 13-ounce can artichoke hearts in water, drained

3 cloves garlic, minced

Salt and black pepper to taste

Raw vegetables for dipping, such as carrots, celery, and cauliflower

1. Preheat the oven to 350°F. In a food processor or blender, combine the cream cheese, ricotta, spinach, Parmesan, artichoke hearts, and garlic. Puree until smooth, scraping down the sides of the bowl as necessary. Season with salt and pepper.

2. Place the artichoke mixture in an ovenproof dish. Bake for about 25 minutes, or until hot and bubbly. Alternatively, use the microwave: Cook in a microwave-safe dish on High for 3 to 4 minutes, rotating the dish one-quarter turn halfway through cooking. Serve immediately with the vegetables. If desired, the dip can also be served at room temperature. (Be sure to taste for seasoning and add more salt and pepper if necessary—cold foods have less flavor than hot.)

Per Serving (¼ cup dip, without vegetables): calories, 80; fat (g), 5; carbohydrates (g), 4; protein (g), 5; cholesterol (mg), 17; sodium (mg), 180.

HEALTH CHECK

• This dish is a great way to incorporate fresh vegetables into your diet and makes snacking on these crunchy treats very tasty.

• This is a good low-calorie recipe for those trying to avoid weight gain.

• Replacing whole-milk cheeses with low-fat versions cuts fat and cholesterol, thus preventing weight gain and reducing the risk of heart disease—always a concern for smokers.

CHAPTER 13
Soups

There's nothing better to calm your nerves than a delicious bowl of hot, steaming soup. A pot of flavorful broth, stocked with vegetables, meats, or seafood, is also a great way to replenish your stores of vitamins and minerals, which smokers often lack. If you once relied on cigarettes to reduce tension, you'll find that sipping on a hot cup of tasty soup in a pleasant setting can have a similarly quieting, soothing effect.

These homemade soups are designed to be low in fat without compromising flavor or body. Keep them on hand as a great low-calorie meal during your early weeks of quitting smoking. If you feel your weight creeping up, and the scale confirms it, make a pot of Creamy Vegetable Soup (page 173), Gazpacho (page 175), or Tomato and Basil Soup (page 180). A good-sized bowl will fill you right up, with relatively few calories.

CORN CHOWDER

SERVES 4

*T*here's nothing more satisfying than a bowl of hot soup on a cold day, and this corn-studded chowder fits the bill well. Hearty and filling, this soup is great with a piece of crusty bread for dipping.

2 teaspoons olive oil

1 medium onion, coarsely chopped

1 10-ounce package thawed frozen corn kernels

2 cups low-fat, low-sodium chicken broth

1 large russet potato (about 13

ounces), baked, peeled, and diced

½ teaspoon ground cumin

½ teaspoon ground coriander

½ teaspoon chili powder

1 cup nonfat milk

Salt and black pepper to taste

1. In a large, heavy, nonstick saucepan, heat the oil over medium-low heat. Add the onion and cook for about 3 minutes, or until slightly softened. Add the corn kernels and cook for 3 minutes more. Add 1 cup of the chicken broth, the potato, cumin, coriander, and chili powder. Stir with a wooden spoon for 3 minutes, or until well blended and warmed through.

2. Pour half the mixture into a food processor or blender and puree until smooth. Return the pureed mixture to the pan and stir in the remaining chicken broth. Partially cover the pan and bring the soup to a slow boil. Reduce the heat and simmer for 10 minutes, stirring occasionally.

3. Stir in the milk, salt, and pepper and simmer for 3 to 4 minutes more, until heated through. Serve immediately.

Per Serving (1 cup): calories, 170; fat (g), 4; carbohydrates (g), 29; protein (g), 7; cholesterol (mg), 4; sodium (mg), 170.

HEALTH CHECK

• When you're craving a high-carbohydrate food, your body may need serotonin, one of the brain chemicals that smoking stimulates. Corn is one of those starchy foods that will help raise the serotonin level in your brain and thus calm you without the need to smoke.

• Using nonfat milk instead of half-and-half saves 7 grams of fat and 80 calories per serving.

• Corn is a good source of vitamin A, which is often low in the blood of smokers.

CREAMY VEGETABLE SOUP

SERVES 2 (4 CUPS)

*M*aking a nice vegetable soup is the perfect way to increase your intake of vitamins and minerals and at the same time use up those perishable items in your refrigerator. I prefer using one type of vegetable, but you can mix and match. Try broccoli, asparagus, cauliflower, or even celery—one of my all-time favorites. Simply combine your choice of vegetable with chicken broth, season with a bit of onion (unless you're using onion as a base), garlic, salt, and pepper, and discover an incredibly easy soup that tastes amazingly creamy, considering it has no cream.

2 teaspoons olive oil

½ medium onion, coarsely chopped

½ pound vegetable of choice, roughly chopped (asparagus, broccoli, cauliflower, celery, etc.)

1 clove garlic, thinly sliced

3½ cups low-fat, low-sodium chicken broth

Salt and black pepper to taste

1. In a large, heavy saucepan, heat the oil over medium heat. Add the onion, vegetable of choice, and garlic and cook for about 7 minutes, or until softened.
2. Add the chicken broth and bring to a boil. Reduce the heat, partially cover the pan, and simmer gently for 45 minutes.
3. Transfer the soup to a blender or food processor and puree, in batches if necessary, until smooth and velvety. Return to the pan, season with the salt and pepper, and bring back to a slow simmer before serving.

Per Serving (2 cups): calories, 130; fat (g), 6; carbohydrates (g), 15; protein (g), 10; cholesterol (mg), 9; sodium (mg), 360.

HEALTH CHECK
• Broccoli and cauliflower are from the cruciferous family of vegetables, which studies have shown help protect against cancer.
• This dish calls for olive oil, which is primarily a monounsaturated fat that helps reduce cholesterol—an important goal for smokers, who are at a greater risk for heart disease.

FRENCH ONION SOUP

I like to make a meal of this classic comfort dish of onions, broth, bread, and cheese. My version has been updated by cutting back on the cheese and the oil. Don't try to rush the onions—long, slow cooking creates this soup's characteristic rich flavor.

1 tablespoon canola oil
1½ pounds yellow onions, very thinly sliced
1½ tablespoons all-purpose flour
4 cups water or low-fat, low-sodium chicken broth, or a combination

Salt and black pepper to taste
6 very thin slices baguette (about 2 ounces), lightly toasted
2 ounces Gruyère or Swiss cheese, grated (about ½ cup)

1. In a large nonstick skillet, heat the oil over low heat. Add the onions and cook very slowly for 45 minutes, until softened and browned, stirring often.
2. Add the flour and stir for 3 to 4 minutes, taking care not to allow it to scorch. Add the water, salt, and pepper, stir thoroughly, and bring to a simmer. Partially cover the pan and cook for about 20 minutes more, or until thickened.
3. Position the broiler rack about 8 inches below the heat source and preheat the broiler. Ladle the soup into ovenproof bowls and top each with a slice of the toasted bread. Scatter the grated cheese over the bread, then place the bowls under the broiler for 2 to 3 minutes, until the cheese is bubbling and brown. Serve immediately.

Per Serving (¾ cup soup, with bread and cheese): calories, 150; fat (g), 7; carbohydrates (g), 17; protein (g), 7; cholesterol (mg), 13; sodium (mg), 200.

HEALTH CHECK
• This version has only 7 grams of fat per serving, half to a third that of traditional French onion soup.
• This recipe calls for very little cheese, thus keeping the calorie count low, but it still provides enough fat for flavor and satisfaction.

GAZPACHO

SERVES 4

*T*hese freshly blended vegetables are full of vibrant, robust flavor. Make a batch and enjoy it right away, and over the course of two or three days. The optional olive oil adds 2 grams of fat and 20 calories to each serving.

5 medium ripe tomatoes, seeded and chopped

3 small cucumbers, peeled, seeded, and chopped

2 small green bell peppers, seeded and chopped

1 small red bell pepper, seeded and chopped

1 small red onion, chopped

3 cups tomato juice

3 tablespoons balsamic vinegar

2 tablespoons fresh lemon juice

2 cloves garlic, minced

Dash of hot pepper sauce

Salt and black pepper to taste

2 teaspoons olive oil, for serving (optional)

1. Reserve ½ cup each of the tomatoes, cucumbers, and green peppers for the garnish. In a blender, combine the remaining tomatoes, cucumbers, and green peppers with the red pepper, onion, tomato juice, balsamic vinegar, lemon juice, garlic, pepper sauce, salt, and pepper. Puree the mixture until smooth, scraping down the sides of the pitcher as necessary. Cover and refrigerate until well chilled (or up to 3 days).

2. Combine the reserved tomatoes, cucumbers, and green peppers in a bowl. Ladle the soup into chilled bowls and top each with a generous scoop of the mixed vegetables. Drizzle each serving with ½ teaspoon of olive oil, if desired, and sprinkle with more black pepper.

Per Serving (1½ cups): calories, 140; fat (g), 1; carbohydrates (g), 32; protein (g), 5; cholesterol (mg), 0; sodium (mg), 750.

HEALTH CHECK

• Vegetables add a shot of vitamins C and A, antioxidants that studies have shown help destroy the process that creates cancer cells.

• Fresh vegetables and seasonings offer an exciting zip for new ex-smokers whose taste buds are just waking up.

• This cold soup provides a cool, soothing feeling in the back of the throat, and will help to calm the nerves during tough times.

HOME-ALONE CHICKEN SOUP

SERVES 1

*M*ade from the simplest ingredients that you might already have on hand, this recipe is perfect if you or someone in your home is feeling under the weather, or simply need a little TLC at the end of a busy day. It's not only soothing, it's also one of the tastiest recipes I've ever created.

1½ cups low-fat, low-sodium
  chicken broth
1 clove garlic, finely chopped
¼ cup of your favorite uncooked
  noodles or macaroni

1 teaspoon fresh lemon juice
Black pepper to taste

1. In a small saucepan, combine the chicken broth and garlic. Bring to a boil over medium heat. Add the noodles and cook for about 8 minutes more, or until they are tender.
2. When the noodles are done, stir in the lemon juice and black pepper and serve at once.

Per Serving: calories, 140; fat (g), 3.5; carbohydrates (g), 23; protein (g), 8; cholesterol (mg), 8; sodium (mg), 170.

HEALTH CHECK
• When you're craving a high-carbohydrate food, your body may need serotonin. The pasta will help raise the serotonin level in your brain and calm you down, much like a cigarette used to do in the old days.
• Lemon juice adds a little zip to food that new ex-smokers, with their newly awakened taste buds, will appreciate.

SPICY LENTIL SOUP

SERVES 4

*T*he secret ingredient in this easy soup is salsa, which adds a spicy flavor without being too hot. Lentils cook more quickly than many other legumes, in about 20 minutes, so they're great for a same-day soup. Of course, you can also make this recipe ahead of time to enjoy on an unexpectedly cold night.

1 cup brown lentils, rinsed and picked over

2½ cups water

2 cups low-fat, low-sodium chicken broth

2 medium carrots, coarsely chopped

1 medium onion, coarsely chopped

1 cup fresh or bottled tomato salsa

Salt and black pepper to taste

2 tablespoons grated Parmesan cheese, for serving (optional)

1. In a large saucepan, combine the lentils, water, broth, carrots, onion, and salsa. Bring the mixture to a boil over high heat.

2. Cover the pan and reduce the heat so that the mixture simmers very gently. Cook for 40 minutes, or until the lentils are tender and the soup is quite thick, stirring occasionally. Season with the salt and pepper. Serve in warmed soup bowls, sprinkled with grated Parmesan, if desired.

• **VARIATION:** To make a thicker soup, transfer about one-quarter of the mixture to a blender or food processor and blend until smooth. Return to the pan and stir thoroughly. Heat through before serving.

Per Serving (1¼ cups): calories, 225; fat (g), 2; carbohydrates (g), 40; protein (g), 17; cholesterol (mg), 3; sodium (mg), 380.

HEALTH CHECK

• When you're craving a high-carbohydrate food, your body may need serotonin. Lentils are a starchy food that will help raise the serotonin level in your brain and calm you down.

• Lentils give a boost of fiber with relatively few calories, creating the sense of feeling full without a lot of fat.

• Lentils are an excellent source of folic acid, which is generally lacking in smokers' diets. In addition, folic acid is especially important for pregnant women, or for those who intend to become pregnant, to prevent birth defects.

SEAFOOD GUMBO

SERVES 8

*T*his light version of traditional gumbo—which still packs a wallop of flavor—is a lot healthier than the original. Browning the flour accomplishes two things: It adds extra flavor and thickens the soup at the same time.

½ cup all-purpose flour

6 cups low-fat, low-sodium chicken broth

2 teaspoons canola oil

4 cloves garlic, finely chopped

2 medium onions, finely chopped

2 stalks celery, finely chopped

1 small red bell pepper, seeded and finely chopped

1 medium tomato, seeded and chopped

1 bay leaf

¼ teaspoon dried thyme

¼ teaspoon dried oregano

¼ teaspoon paprika

¼ teaspoon black pepper

Pinch each of salt, cayenne pepper, and crushed red pepper flakes

¾ pound medium raw shrimp, peeled and deveined

4 cups hot cooked white or brown rice, for serving

1. Heat a large nonstick skillet over low heat and add the flour. Cook until golden brown, stirring constantly to prevent scorching, for about 15 minutes. Remove from the heat and set aside.

2. In a medium saucepan, bring the chicken broth to a boil. Reduce the heat to very low and cover the pan.

3. In a large saucepan, heat the oil over medium-high heat. Add the garlic, onions, celery, bell pepper, and tomato and cook for about 10 minutes, or until the vegetables are soft, stirring often. Stir in the bay leaf, thyme, oregano, paprika, pepper, salt, cayenne, and red pepper flakes. Continue cooking for 3 to 4 minutes, until the herbs are fragrant. Add the shrimp and cook for about 3 minutes, or until they are pink and firm.

4. Gradually add the browned flour, 1 tablespoon at a time, stirring to combine with the shrimp mixture. Gradually add the warm chicken stock, one

cup at a time, stirring constantly. The liquid will start to thicken. Bring the mixture to a slow boil, cover the pan, and reduce the heat. Simmer for 30 minutes, stirring occasionally. Serve immediately over hot rice.

Per Serving (2 cups gumbo, without rice): calories, 270; fat (g), 7; carbohydrates (g), 29; protein (g), 26; cholesterol (mg), 140; sodium (mg), 320.

HEALTH CHECK

• This updated gumbo saves 10 grams of fat and about 100 calories per serving when compared to a traditional recipe.

• Although a serving of shrimp contains 173 milligrams of cholesterol, the cholesterol is offset by the low level of saturated fat in shrimp: only .2 grams, or 1 gram total fat per 3-ounce serving.

TOMATO AND BASIL SOUP

SERVES 4

*D*on't be intimidated by homemade soups; their flavor is far beyond that of any canned variety. Soup can provide a low-calorie, filling way to round out a meal. The fresh basil and garlic make this one a real winner, and best of all it freezes well. Dried basil cannot be substituted for fresh.

1 tablespoon olive oil	1 teaspoon dried rosemary
1 28-ounce can whole tomatoes	½ teaspoon salt
1 medium onion, chopped	½ cup tightly packed fresh basil
6 cloves garlic, chopped	leaves, coarsely chopped
1 cup water	(chop at the last minute;
½ cup canned tomato puree	otherwise they'll turn black)
1 tablespoon sugar	

1. In a large skillet, heat the olive oil over high heat. Add the tomatoes with their liquid, onion, and garlic and bring to a boil, breaking up the tomatoes with the back of a spoon. Reduce the heat and simmer for 5 minutes, or until the onion is softened.
2. Add the water, tomato puree, sugar, rosemary, and salt and blend well. Return to a simmer and cook for 12 minutes, stirring often.
3. Transfer the mixture, in batches if necessary, to a blender or food processor and blend until smooth. Return to the pan, stir in the basil, and heat through before serving. If desired, cool completely and freeze for up to 6 months.

Per Serving (1 cup): calories, 125; fat (g), 4; carbohydrates (g), 22; protein (g), 4; cholesterol (mg), 0; sodium (mg), 450.

HEALTH CHECK
• With only 125 calories per serving, this summery soup is a good value for those trying to avoid weight gain.
• Lots of fresh basil and garlic add flavor without adding fat or calories. This will wake up those drowsy taste buds!
• Tomatoes add a shot of vitamin B_6, which is generally lacking in smokers' diets.

VEGETABLE SOUP

SERVES 6

When one of my patients has been steadily losing weight, and then reaches a plateau and can't seem to lose more, I suggest this recipe. Make a batch on the weekend, then have a bowl for a weekday lunch or dinner— you'll have a filling and satisfying meal that is low in calories. The soup will keep for up to five days, covered and chilled. Reheat the soup, thinning with water as needed, since it may thicken after being chilled.

1 tablespoon olive oil

½ pound lean turkey ham, chopped

2 medium onions, chopped

2 large carrots, cut into ½-inch dice

2 stalks celery, cut into ½-inch dice

3 cloves garlic, finely chopped

2 medium zucchini, cut into ½-inch dice

¼ pound fresh green beans, trimmed and cut into ½-inch

pieces, or 1½ cups thawed frozen cut green beans

½ pound boiling potatoes, peeled and cut into ½-inch dice

4 cups shredded green cabbage (preferably Savoy)

1 28-ounce can whole tomatoes, drained well and coarsely chopped

4½ cups low-fat, low-sodium chicken broth

¼ cup freshly grated Parmesan cheese, for serving

1. In a large, heavy saucepan or soup pot, heat the oil over medium heat. Add the turkey ham and cook for about 4 minutes, stirring, or until crisp and pale golden. Add the onions and cook for 4 minutes, stirring, or until softened. Add the carrots, celery, and garlic and cook the mixture, still stirring, for 4 minutes more. As you are cooking the vegetables, add a little water or broth if the mixture seems very dry or in danger of scorching.

2. Add the zucchini, green beans, and potatoes and cook, stirring, for 4 minutes. Add the cabbage and continue cooking until it is wilted. Stir in

the tomatoes and chicken broth and bring the soup to a slow boil. Cover the pan, reduce the heat, and simmer the soup for 1 hour.

3. Serve the soup in warmed bowls, sprinkled with grated Parmesan.

Per Serving (1½ cups): calories, 230; fat (g), 6; carbohydrates (g), 32; protein (g), 16; cholesterol (mg), 34; sodium (mg), 840.

HEALTH CHECK

• Vegetables, especially green beans and root vegetables such as carrots, add a boost of fiber to the system. Fiber gives you a sense of fullness without excessive calorie intake, and will satisfy a craving safely.

• This combination of vegetables contributes vitamins A and C plus beta carotene— all antioxidants that help prevent the onset of cancer and heart disease.

• The chemical galanin may be responsible for our cravings for fat. (See page 44.) This soup has just enough fat to satisfy the urge without a calorie or fat overload.

CHAPTER 14
Salads

Adding a side salad to your meal, or even making a meal out of a salad by adding some protein, is a good bet for the new ex-smoker who is trying to watch his or her calorie intake. You not only get a considerable volume of food, but a vivid contrast of flavors and textures as well. To the reawakening taste buds of the new ex-smoker, this combination makes for an exciting meal. To build in some added control over how much of the main course you eat, particularly with carbohydrate-rich pizza or pasta, including a salad will help fill you up before you overdo it. For side salads, I suggest the Basic Green Salad with Vinaigrette (page 194), Chopped Cucumber-Tomato Salad (page 189), Crunchy Cucumber Slices (page 190), or Wilted Spinach Salad (page 200).

Other salads are a meal in themselves. One of my favorites is the Chinese Chicken Salad (page 187), which is likely to become a favorite of yours too. The Barbecued Chicken Chopped Salad (page 185) and the Meatless Taco Salad (page 195) also make great one-dish meals.

For a simple lunch at home, try the apple and cucumber salad (page 184)—chop up one of each, add a bit of yogurt and cilantro, and you're done! If your entrée is fish or chicken, choose one of the heartier salads, such as the Warm Potato Salad (page 197) or the White Bean Salad (page 198). With all of these salads, you'll transcend the old stigma of salads as a punishing diet food. Best of all, eating salads will help increase your intake of vegetables without adding significant fat. That's a primary objective for anyone trying to manage their weight.

APPLE, CUCUMBER, AND CILANTRO SALAD

SERVES 2

*T*he key to this delicious dish is a firm, sweet red apple. There is no need to peel it, but do so if you wish.

1 large Red Delicious apple, cored and cut into ½-inch dice

1 cucumber, peeled, halved lengthwise, seeded, and cut into ½-inch dice

1 tablespoon light mayonnaise

1 tablespoon finely chopped fresh cilantro

¼ teaspoon salt

In a large bowl, combine the apple, cucumber, mayonnaise, cilantro, and salt. Toss to mix and serve, or cover tightly and refrigerate for up to 1 day.

Per Serving (1 cup): calories, 110; fat (g), 3; carbohydrates (g), 21; protein (g), 1; cholesterol (mg), 0; sodium (mg), 330.

HEALTH CHECK

• Fresh fruits and vegetables give a boost of fiber with relatively few calories, a great alternative when you're tempted to reach for a cigarette.

• Light mayonnaise replaces regular mayonnaise, representing a savings of about 3 grams fat and nearly 30 calories per serving.

• The apple and cucumber provide a crunch that satisfies the need for oral gratification.

BARBECUED CHICKEN CHOPPED SALAD

SERVES 4

*T*his is a popular salad in restaurants lately, and I've lightened it up without compromising the great flavor.

4 cooked boneless, skinless chicken breast halves (about 1 pound), cut into ½-inch cubes

¼ cup plus 2 tablespoons barbecue sauce

¼ cup fat-free ranch dressing

8 cups chopped lettuce, such as romaine

1 15-ounce can black beans, drained

2 cups thawed frozen corn

½ medium jicama, peeled and diced

½ medium red onion, finely chopped

1 cup coarsely chopped fresh cilantro

1. In a medium bowl, combine the chicken with ¼ cup of the barbecue sauce, toss to coat, and set aside. In a small bowl, mix together the remaining 2 tablespoons barbecue sauce and the ranch dressing and set aside.

2. In a large bowl, combine the lettuce, beans, corn, jicama, red onion, and cilantro and toss together gently. Add just enough of the ranch-barbecue dressing mixture to coat the ingredients, and toss again gently.

3. Divide the lettuce mixture evenly among serving plates and top with the chicken mixture. Serve immediately.

Per Serving (2½ cups): calories, 375; fat (g), 3; carbohydrates (g), 50; protein (g), 39; cholesterol (mg), 66; sodium (mg), 820.

HEALTH CHECK

• This tangy dressing will delight new ex-smokers whose taste buds are waking up. It tastes sinful but isn't.

• Fresh vegetables give a boost of fiber and crunch with relatively few calories.

• The protein in chicken increases the feeling of fullness, so you eat less and feel full longer.

CHICKEN SALAD WITH APPLE
SERVES 4

*T*he apple and celery add crunch and flavor to this salad; you could also add half a teaspoon of curry powder to the light mayonnaise for an exotic Indian flair. It keeps well in the refrigerator for a day or two and, when stuffed into a pita pocket, turns a brown-bag lunch into a gourmet treat. You can also turn this into an entrée by serving it on a bed of salad greens. Alternatively, double the recipe for a buffet table.

¼ cup light mayonnaise
1 tablespoon whole-grain
   mustard
1 teaspoon fresh lemon juice
Salt and black pepper to taste
4 cooked boneless, skinless
   chicken breast halves, cut into
   ½-inch dice (or half the meat
   from a 3-pound roast chicken,
   diced, see page 214)

1 stalk celery, cut into ¼-inch
   dice
¼ medium onion, cut into ¼-
   inch dice
1 small apple, peeled, cored,
   and diced
1 tablespoon finely chopped
   fresh cilantro

1. In a large bowl, whisk together the mayonnaise, mustard, and lemon juice. If desired, thin with water to a coating consistency. Whisk in the salt and pepper.

2. Fold in the diced chicken, celery, onion, apple, and cilantro and taste for seasoning.

3. Mound the salad onto a chilled platter and serve immediately, or cover and refrigerate.

Per Serving (1 cup): calories, 210; fat (g), 7; carbohydrates (g), 9; protein (g), 27; cholesterol (mg), 66; sodium (mg), 310.

HEALTH CHECK
- Though it contains only 6 grams of fat per serving, this salad is jumping with flavor.
- Apple and celery provide a crunch that satisfies the need for oral gratification.
- With only 210 calories per serving, this salad is a good value for those trying to avoid weight gain.

CHINESE CHICKEN SALAD

SERVES 4

*M*y friend Hillary Jaye came up with this take on Chinese chicken salad, and it's sure to become a regular in your repertoire. She took the standard lettuce, chicken, and dressing formula and spruced it up with fresh mint, cilantro, and ginger. The result is infinitely more flavorful and healthful than any version you are likely to encounter at a restaurant. Reserve a little for your lunch the next day, and add the dressing when you're ready to eat to keep the salad fresh and crunchy. The longer you let the dressing stand, the more it becomes infused with the ginger and the tastier it gets.

DRESSING
½ cup seasoned rice wine vinegar
1 teaspoon sugar
½ teaspoon olive oil
½ teaspoon sesame oil
½ teaspoon low-sodium soy sauce
2 teaspoons finely minced fresh ginger

SALAD
1 tablespoon low-sodium soy sauce
1 tablespoon sesame oil
1 pound boneless, skinless chicken breasts
Black pepper to taste

½ pound mixed baby salad greens or chopped lettuce, such as romaine or butter
¼ pound fresh bean sprouts
½ cup (packed) chopped fresh cilantro
3 green onions (scallions), thinly sliced
½ cup (packed) chopped fresh mint leaves
1 medium red bell pepper, seeded and cut into ½-inch dice
1 teaspoon sesame seeds, for garnish

1. To make the dressing: In a small bowl, combine the vinegar, sugar, olive oil, sesame oil, soy sauce, and minced ginger. Whisk together thoroughly and set aside at room temperature while preparing the salad.

2. Preheat the oven to 350°F. In an 8-inch square baking dish, combine the soy sauce and sesame oil. Add the chicken breasts and turn to coat all sides evenly. Season with black pepper and bake for 20 to 25 minutes, until the

breasts are firm, slightly golden, and cooked through with no trace of pink remaining, turning after 10 minutes. Remove the pan from the oven and drain any accumulated liquid. Cut the chicken breasts into 1-inch dice.

3. While the chicken is cooking, in a large salad bowl, combine the salad greens, bean sprouts, cilantro, green onions, mint, and bell pepper. Add the diced chicken and the dressing to the lettuce mixture and toss gently to coat well. Sprinkle with the sesame seeds and serve.

Per Serving (2½ cups): calories, 220; fat (g), 4.5; carbohydrates (g), 13; protein (g), 32; cholesterol (mg), 65; sodium (mg), 280.

HEALTH CHECK

• This tangy dressing uses rice wine vinegar, ginger, and a bit of sugar for great taste and lots of zip. New ex-smokers whose taste buds are just getting back to normal will appreciate the wake-up call.

• The protein in chicken acts to increase the feeling of fullness, which means you eat less and feel full longer.

• Vegetables packed with fiber help fill us up quickly.

CHOPPED CUCUMBER-TOMATO SALAD

SERVES 2

*M*arinating in a mix of lemon juice, tomatoes, and capers brings out the wonderful cucumber flavor in this salad. Use it as part of a sandwich construction, or as an accompaniment to grilled or poached fish. No fat at all is necessary in this delicious combination of ingredients.

1 European cucumber, diced, or
  2 medium cucumbers, peeled,
  halved lengthwise, seeded,
  and diced
3 medium plum tomatoes,
  seeded and diced

2 tablespoons capers, rinsed
  and patted dry
1 tablespoon fresh lemon juice
Black pepper to taste

In a large bowl, combine the diced cucumber, tomatoes, capers, lemon juice, and pepper and toss to mix. Cover and refrigerate for 30 minutes before serving.

Per Serving: calories, 15; fat (g), 0; carbohydrates (g), 3; protein (g), 1; cholesterol (mg), 0; sodium (mg), 85.

HEALTH CHECK
- Tomatoes add a shot of vitamin C, which is generally lacking in smokers' diets.
- Fresh vegetables give a boost of fiber with relatively few calories. Fiber provides a feeling of fullness and thus satisfies a craving safely.
- Cucumbers lend a nice crunch that will soothe the need for oral gratification.

CRUNCHY CUCUMBER SLICES

SERVES 2

*T*his is a delicious snack that is both light and low in calories, but certainly packs a punch of flavor. Use half a European cucumber if they're available, since they do not need to be peeled or seeded (one is equal to two regular cucumbers) and you do not lose vitamins and nutrients by removing the skin. I prefer kosher salt, which is not iodized and is therefore less bitter than regular salt.

½ European cucumber or 1 medium cucumber	1 teaspoon kosher salt ½ cup rice wine vinegar

1. If using a regular cucumber, peel, cut in half lengthwise, and remove the seeds. Cut the cucumber on the diagonal into ¼-inch slices. Spread the slices on a paper towel and sprinkle with the salt. Leave to drain for 30 minutes.
2. Thoroughly blot the salt and liquid from the tops of the cucumber slices with more paper towels. Transfer to a small serving bowl, drizzle with the rice vinegar, and toss well. Cover with plastic wrap and refrigerate for 1 hour for the flavors to develop.

Per Serving: calories, 20; fat (g), 0; carbohydrates (g), 4; protein (g), 1; cholesterol (mg), 0; sodium (mg), 270.

HEALTH CHECK
- With only 20 calories and 0 fat grams per serving, this is an ultra-virtuous treat.
- Vinegar adds a little zip for new ex-smokers whose taste buds are just waking up.
- Cucumbers provide a nice crunch that soothes the need for oral gratification.

GRATED VEGETABLE PLATTER WITH VINAIGRETTE

SERVES 8

A health-conscious cook must have a long list of tricks up his or her sleeve for preparing vegetables in new and interesting ways so they're appealing and delicious! One tactic is to cut veggies up in various forms—here they're all grated, which makes a nice presentation alongside a sandwich. Seasoned with the simple but fabulous flavors of the vinaigrette, this salad should entice even those who often pass on vegetables. Sometimes I use only carrots, or carrots and one other vegetable, but if you are having a party this entire array is very festive.

VINAIGRETTE

¼ cup plus 1 tablespoon red wine vinegar

3 tablespoons Dijon mustard

½ cup olive oil

2 tablespoons minced fresh basil or 2 teaspoons dried

2 tablespoons minced fresh chives or green onions (scallions)

Salt and black pepper to taste

SALAD

2 large cucumbers, peeled, halved lengthwise, seeded, and thinly sliced

½ teaspoon salt

2 large raw beets, peeled and grated

2 large carrots, grated

2 large zucchini, grated

1 bunch radishes, trimmed, for garnish

1. To make the vinaigrette: In a small bowl, whisk together the vinegar and Dijon mustard. Gradually whisk in the olive oil until emulsified. Add the basil and chives and season to taste with the salt and pepper. (The vinaigrette can be made 1 day ahead. Cover and refrigerate.)

2. In a large bowl, toss together the cucumbers and salt and let stand for 1 hour. Rinse, drain well, and pat dry with paper towels. Place the cucumbers in a small bowl and add just enough vinaigrette to coat. Toss gently.

3. Place the grated beets, carrots, and zucchini in separate bowls. Toss each vegetable with just enough dressing to coat. (Vegetables can be prepared 4 hours ahead. Cover and chill.)

4. On a large platter, mound each vegetable in a separate pile. Garnish with radishes and serve.

Per Serving: calories, 153; fat (g), 9; carbohydrates (g), 8; protein (g), 2; cholesterol (mg), 0; sodium (mg), 165.

HEALTH CHECK

• Carrots and beets are high in vitamin A, which tends to be lacking in smokers' diets.

• Fresh vegetables give a boost of fiber, which helps fill you up quickly with a low calorie count so you eat less.

• This recipe is low in calories, while still providing enough fat for flavor and satisfaction.

GREEN BEANS VINAIGRETTE

SERVES 2

*I*f you were raised on home-grown, garden-fresh green beans like I was, you'll love this "gussied up" version of green bean salad.

½ pound green beans, trimmed
1 tablespoon rice wine vinegar
2 teaspoons Dijon mustard

½ teaspoon salt
¼ teaspoon black pepper
1 tablespoon olive oil

1. In a medium saucepan, bring a generous amount of lightly salted water to a boil. Add the beans and cook for 4 minutes, then drain and immediately rinse under cold running water to stop the cooking and preserve the color. Shake the beans dry, and then transfer to a medium bowl.

2. In a small bowl, whisk together the vinegar, mustard, salt, and pepper. Whisk in the oil until emulsified.

3. Add the vinaigrette to the beans, toss well to coat, and serve.

Per Serving: calories, 80; fat (g), 5; carbohydrates (g), 9; protein (g), 2; cholesterol (mg), 0; sodium (mg), 670.

HEALTH CHECK

• This recipe contains only 80 calories per serving, a good value for those trying to avoid weight gain.

• Rice wine vinegar adds a nice zip for new ex-smokers whose taste buds are just waking up.

• This recipe calls for very little oil, keeping calories low while still providing enough fat for flavor and satisfaction.

BASIC GREEN SALAD WITH VINAIGRETTE

SERVES 4; MAKES ¼ CUP VINAIGRETTE

*I*t's always helpful to have a great basic salad dressing on hand, and this one fits the bill—it's full of flavor, but not fat. Only a little is needed to dress an average-size salad. Since it's such a simple dressing, this is one place where you may want to splurge on a nice extra-virgin olive oil.

VINAIGRETTE

1 clove garlic, finely chopped

1 tablespoon balsamic vinegar

1 teaspoon fresh lemon juice

½ teaspoon Dijon mustard

¼ teaspoon sugar (optional)

Salt and black pepper to taste

2 tablespoons olive oil,
    preferably extra-virgin

4 cups torn salad greens

1. In a jar with a tight-fitting lid, combine the garlic, vinegar, lemon juice, mustard, sugar, if desired, salt, and pepper. Shake vigorously, then add the oil and shake again until the mixture is emulsified. If desired, refrigerate the vinaigrette for up to 3 days.

2. In a chilled bowl, toss the salad greens with enough vinaigrette just to coat, and serve immediately.

• **VARIATIONS FOR VINAIGRETTE:**

  • Add ½ shallot, minced, or 2 green onions (scallions), white and light green parts only, minced.

  • Add 1 teaspoon minced fresh basil, rosemary, or thyme, or use a scant ½ teaspoon of the dried herb.

  • Add 1 teaspoon anchovy paste or 1 anchovy, minced.

  • Substitute champagne, raspberry, or rice wine vinegar for balsamic.

Per Serving: calories, 60; fat (g), 5; carbohydrates (g), 4; protein (g), 1; cholesterol (mg), 0; sodium (mg), 90.

HEALTH CHECK

• This recipe calls for very little oil, keeping calories low while still providing enough fat for flavor and satisfaction.

• Dark leafy salad greens are packed with fiber, which helps fill you up quickly with very few calories.

MEATLESS TACO SALAD

SERVES 2

*F*orget the heavy, fat-laden taco salads of yore—this is a fresh, crunchy, and yes, meatless, version of the popular salad that is sure to please. I like to top it with some sliced Grilled Chicken Breasts with Beer (see page 00) and serve it with a cold glass of limeade on a warm summer night.

4 cups shredded romaine lettuce (about 1 head)	½ cup bottled mild salsa
1 cup shredded red cabbage	½ cup chopped fresh cilantro
1 cup canned black beans, rinsed and drained	¼ cup nonfat sour cream
1 cup canned corn, rinsed and drained	2 tablespoons pitted sliced black olives

1. In a large bowl, combine the romaine, cabbage, black beans, corn, salsa, and cilantro. Toss together thoroughly.
2. Divide the salad between two plates and top each with a dollop of sour cream and a few olive slices. Serve immediately.

Per Serving: calories, 250; fat (g), 3; carbohydrates (g), 45; protein (g), 14; cholesterol (mg), 0; sodium (mg), 760.

HEALTH CHECK
- Nonfat sour cream replaces regular sour cream and saves about 5 grams of fat and nearly 50 calories per serving.
- This tasty salad has only 3 grams of fat per serving.
- Fresh vegetables are packed with fiber, which helps fill you up quickly with few calories so you eat less.

TOMATO, RED ONION, AND AVOCADO SALAD

SERVES 4

*T*his easy and flavorful salad is a great accompaniment to a sandwich or lean steak such as flank steak.

4 medium tomatoes, diced

1 medium red onion, finely chopped

1 medium ripe avocado, diced

3 tablespoons balsamic vinegar

1 teaspoon olive oil

Salt and black pepper to taste

1. In a medium bowl, combine the tomatoes, red onion, avocado, vinegar, olive oil, and salt and pepper. Toss together gently and chill for 1 hour to allow flavors to meld.

2. Just before serving, toss again to redistribute the dressing. Taste for seasoning, adjust if necessary, and serve.

Per Serving: calories, 135; fat (g), 9; carbohydrates (g), 13; protein (g), 2; cholesterol (mg), 0; sodium (mg), 150.

HEALTH CHECK

• Avocado is a good source of vitamin B_6, which is generally lacking in smokers' diets.

• Balsamic vinegar adds a nice zip for new ex-smokers whose taste buds are waking up. Since it is so mild, you need less oil to balance its tartness.

• This recipe calls for very little oil, keeping calories low while still providing enough fat for flavor and satisfaction.

WARM POTATO SALAD
SERVES 4

I remember asking my mother for her potato salad recipe many years ago. Now she's asking for mine! This is a modern version with great flavor and very little of the fat found in a traditional potato salad. It can be made just before serving, or prepared a day in advance and refrigerated.

1 pound red potatoes, peeled
  and cut into ½-inch cubes
Salt and black pepper to taste
1 tablespoon extra-virgin olive
  oil

1 large onion, thinly sliced
¼ cup rice wine vinegar
1 tablespoon sugar

1. Place the potatoes in a large saucepan, cover them with cold water, and add a little salt. Bring to a boil, reduce the heat, and simmer for about 10 minutes, or until the potatoes are tender but not mushy. Drain well and set aside.
2. In a large cast-iron or nonstick skillet, heat the olive oil over medium-low heat. Add the onion and cook for 5 to 10 minutes, until softened. Season with salt and pepper and add the vinegar and sugar.
3. Increase the heat to medium and scrape all the flavorful bits from the bottom of the pan into the liquid. Cook, stirring, until most of the liquid has evaporated, then add the potatoes and stir them gently, taking care not to break them up into a mush. Serve warm or at room temperature.

Per Serving (¾ cup): calories, 160; fat (g), 4; carbohydrates (g), 30; protein (g), 3; cholesterol (mg), 0; sodium (mg), 75.

HEALTH CHECK
• A complex carbohydrate, potatoes help raise the level of serotonin in the blood and thus go a long way toward pacifying the urge for nicotine.
• Potatoes also add a boost of vitamin C, which is often lacking in smokers' diets.
• This updated version of potato salad saves 11 grams of fat and about 110 calories per serving as compared to a traditional mayonnaise-based recipe.

WHITE BEAN SALAD

SERVES 6

*B*eans provide a good amount of protein without fat, plus complex carbohydrates to keep blood sugars stable. This salad will keep for a day or two in the refrigerator—the flavor actually improves over time. I like to pack it in my lunch during the week; it's also a great item on a buffet table.

1 pound dried white beans, such as navy or lima, rinsed and soaked in water to cover for at least 6 hours, or overnight

2 teaspoons salt

1 tablespoon olive oil

1 cup finely chopped onion

½ medium red bell pepper, seeded and diced (about ½ cup)

½ cup currants or raisins soaked in hot water for 10 minutes, then drained

½ cup white wine vinegar

1½ tablespoons fresh thyme leaves, chopped, or 1 scant tablespoon dried, crumbled

Salt and black pepper to taste

1. Drain the beans and place them in a large, heavy saucepan. Add enough fresh cold water to cover the beans by about 2 inches and bring to a simmer. Cover the pan and simmer for 1 hour.

2. Add the salt, cover again, and simmer for about 30 minutes more, or until the beans are tender but not mushy. (Cooking time will vary with the age of the beans, so this is only a guideline.) Drain the beans and set aside.

3. Heat the olive oil in a large cast-iron or heavy nonstick skillet over medium heat. Add the onion and cook for about 5 minutes, or until softened. Add the red pepper and cook, stirring, for 2 minutes more.

4. Gently stir in the currants, vinegar, thyme, and salt, pepper, and beans. Remove from the heat and let the mixture cool to room temperature. Cover and refrigerate overnight, if possible, for the flavors to develop. Before

serving, bring back to room temperature, taste for seasoning, and add more salt and pepper if necessary.

Per Serving (1 cup): calories, 330; fat (g), 3; carbohydrates (g), 61; protein (g), 17; cholesterol (mg), 0; sodium (mg), 780.

HEALTH CHECK

• The complex carbohydrates in the beans increase serotonin in the brain, giving a calming effect.

• This recipe contains only 3 grams of fat per serving.

• The protein in beans will help keep blood sugars stable well into the day, and thus keep hunger in check.

WILTED SPINACH SALAD

SERVES 4

This spinach salad skips the bacon, but you'll never miss it in this flavor-ful dish. The high vitamin A content naturally present in spinach is a bonus.

DRESSING
1 teaspoon balsamic vinegar
½ teaspoon fresh lemon juice
⅛ teaspoon salt
1 clove garlic, finely chopped
2 tablespoons canola oil
½ teaspoon sugar

SALAD
1 bunch fresh spinach, stemmed
4 green onions (scallions), white and light green parts only, thinly sliced
½ pound mushrooms, thinly sliced
Freshly ground black pepper to taste

1. To make the dressing: In a small, microwave-safe bowl, whisk together the vinegar, lemon juice, salt, sugar, and garlic. Add the oil in a thin stream, whisking all the time, until the dressing is emulsified.

2. In a large salad bowl, combine the spinach, green onions, and mushrooms, and toss together gently.

3. Just before serving, heat the dressing in the microwave on High for 10 to 20 seconds, until hot but not boiling. Pour the dressing over the salad and immediately toss together to slightly wilt the greens. Sprinkle with freshly ground pepper and serve.

Per Serving (1 cup): calories, 70; fat (g), 4; carbohydrates (g), 7; protein (g), 3; cholesterol (mg), 0; sodium (mg), 125.

HEALTH CHECK

• Spinach provides vitamin A as well as folic acid, both of which are generally lacking in smokers' diets. Folic acid is especially important for pregnant women or those who intend to become pregnant because it helps to prevent birth defects.

• This tangy dressing adds a nice zip for new ex-smokers whose taste buds are waking up without packing too much fat.

• Fresh vegetables give a boost of fiber with relatively few calories, thus giving you a sense of fullness that will last.

CHAPTER 15
Main Courses:
Fish, Chicken,
Lean Meats

A tasty, well-prepared main dish often provides all the excitement in the meal. Here you'll find some traditional entrées that have been modified to meet the Personal Nutrition Management Plan criteria while preserving all the flavorful essence of your old favorites. Feasting on such delicious dishes as Oven-Fried Chicken (page 212), Old-Fashioned Beef Stew (page 225), and Best Grilled Swordfish (page 202), you won't feel deprived for a moment.

Protein is one of the building blocks of good nutrition, and it helps to give you a sense of fullness during a meal. Try to feature a protein food as your main course and then add a side dish of vegetables and rice, pasta, a pizza crust, or beans. Choose your vegetables first and your starch second, because starches are much higher in calories than vegetables. Increasing the ratio of vegetables to starch on your plate is the best way to manage calories. For example, depending on your calorie need, you may want to limit rice or pasta to ½ cup and have 1 cup of vegetables or even more. See the Menu Plans beginning on page 80 for examples.

Again, if you once relied on cigarettes to reduce tension, you'll find that eating a wonderful dinner in a pleasant setting can also have a quieting, calming effect.

BEST GRILLED SWORDFISH

SERVES 4

*W*hen you have time to marinate, this is the best way I've found to enhance the flavor of fish. Putting the fish in a plastic bag makes cleanup easy, and the marinating even more efficient. You can substitute any firm white fish for the swordfish, such as halibut, orange roughy, or sea bass. Any leftover will make a great sandwich, taco, or burrito the next day.

⅓ cup fresh lemon juice

3 large cloves garlic, finely chopped

½ cup fresh cilantro sprigs, chopped (optional)

1 tablespoon olive oil

2 pounds swordfish or other firm white fish steaks

Salt and black pepper to taste

1. In a large Ziploc freezer bag, combine the lemon juice, garlic, cilantro, if desired, and olive oil. Seal the bag and shake to mix.

2. Add the fish, reseal, and shake carefully to coat. Marinate in the refrigerator for at least 1 hour, or overnight.

3. Prepare the grill (medium-high heat) or preheat the broiler. If using a grill, be sure to oil the rack so the fish will not stick. Place the fish on the hot grill or under the broiler and cook for 4 to 5 minutes per side (a general guideline is to cook fish for a total of 10 minutes per inch of thickness, or until the fish is firm to the touch and opaque throughout. Season with salt and pepper and serve immediately.

Per Serving: calories, 245; fat (g), 10; carbohydrates (g), 3; protein (g), 34; cholesterol (mg), 66; sodium (mg), 220.

HEALTH CHECK

• Oily fish contains omega-3 fatty acids, which act like biological antifreeze to keep arteries from clogging, thus preventing heart disease, always a concern for smokers.

• The chemical galanin may be responsible for our fat cravings (see page 44). This swordfish recipe has just enough fat to satisfy a craving without a calorie overload.

• This dish calls for olive oil, which is primarily a monounsaturated fat and helps reduce cholesterol, a goal for smokers who are at a greater risk for heart disease and stroke.

BROILED SALMON WITH GARLIC
SERVES 2

*T*his is a great last-minute supper for your recipe repertoire. Just pick up the salmon on your way home from work, and with minimal preparation you'll have a fabulous dinner in less than 15 minutes. Now, that's fast food!

2 salmon fillets (6 ounces each)	**1 teaspoon olive oil**
3 cloves garlic, thinly sliced	**Salt and black pepper to taste**

1. Preheat the broiler and cover a broiling pan with aluminum foil.
2. With a paring knife, make several slits in one side of each salmon fillet and push the sliced garlic into them. Brush both sides of the salmon with olive oil and season with the salt and pepper.
3. Place the salmon on the foil and cook for about 5 minutes. Turn carefully and cook for 5 minutes more, or until the fish is firm to the touch and opaque throughout. (Keep in mind that fish usually cooks at 10 minutes per inch of thickness.) Serve immediately.

Per Serving: calories, 225; fat (g), 8; carbohydrates (g), 2; protein (g), 34; cholesterol (mg), 89; sodium (mg), 115.

HEALTH CHECK
• The protein in fish will help keep blood sugars stable well into the evening, and thus keep hunger in check.
• This dish calls for olive oil, which is primarily a monounsaturated fat and helps reduce cholesterol, a goal for smokers who are at a greater risk for heart disease and stroke.
• Oily fish contains omega-3 fatty acids, which act like biological antifreeze to keep arteries from clogging, thus preventing heart disease, always a concern for smokers.

GRILLED FISH WITH TOMATO SALSA

SERVES 4; MAKES 1½ CUPS SALSA

*T*he combination of fish and fresh salsa makes a quick, delicious, and spicy dish. Serve this salsa with rice or beans; you can change the amounts of the ingredients to suit your own taste, or just use your favorite store-bought salsa if you're short on time. Salsa is best on the day that it's made, but it can be covered and refrigerated for up to two days.

SALSA

½ pound plum tomatoes, seeded and cut into ½-inch dice

½ small onion, cut into ½-inch dice (about ⅓ cup)

2 tablespoons finely chopped fresh cilantro

2 teaspoons fresh lemon juice

¼ fresh serrano chili, stemmed, seeded, and minced

Salt and black pepper to taste

4 white fish steaks, such as halibut or swordfish (about 1½ pounds)

1. To make the salsa: In a medium bowl or container, combine the tomatoes, onion, cilantro, lemon juice, chili, salt, and pepper and toss together until evenly mixed. Set aside.

2. Prepare the grill (medium-high heat) or preheat the broiler. If using a grill, be sure to oil the rack so the fish will not stick.

3. Season the fish by rubbing both sides with a little salt and pepper. Place on the hot grill or under the broiler and cook until the fish is firm to the touch and opaque throughout, turning halfway through the cooking time. (Fish usually cooks at about 10 minutes per inch of thickness.) Divide the fish among plates and top each serving with a spoonful of the salsa. Serve immediately.

Per Serving: calories, 205; fat (g), 4; carbohydrates (g), 4; protein (g), 36; cholesterol (mg), 54; sodium (mg), 230.

HEALTH CHECK

• This recipe has only 4 grams of fat per serving.

• Tomatoes provide a shot of vitamin C, which is generally lacking in smokers' diets.

• Calorie per calorie, protein gives a greater sense of fullness than an equal amount of carbohydrate, so eating fish should allow you to eat fewer calories and feel full longer.

SHRIMP WITH GARLIC AND LEMON

SERVES 6

A good shrimp dish is always a treat, and this simple combination of flavor-enhancing ingredients makes the shellfish taste superb. Plain rice is the perfect accompaniment.

1 teaspoon olive oil

30 medium shrimp (about 1 pound), peeled and deveined if necessary

1 to 2 cloves garlic, finely chopped

Finely chopped zest of ½ lemon

2 tablespoons fresh lemon juice

Salt and black pepper to taste

2 tablespoons finely chopped fresh parsley (optional)

1. In a large, heavy nonstick or cast-iron skillet, heat the olive oil over medium-high heat. Add the shrimp, garlic, and lemon zest and cook for 2 to 3 minutes, tossing occasionally, until the shrimp are firm and pink (do not overcook). Add a teaspoon or two of water if needed to prevent the garlic from burning.

2. Remove the pan from the heat, immediately add the lemon juice, and swirl to mix. Season with the salt and pepper, sprinkle with the parsley, if desired, and serve immediately. Alternatively, serve the dish at room temperature, or cover and refrigerate for up to 12 hours and serve chilled.

Per Serving: calories, 135; fat (g), 3; carbohydrates (g), 2; protein (g), 23; cholesterol (mg), 173; sodium (mg), 300.

HEALTH CHECK

• This dish calls for olive oil, which is primarily a monounsaturated fat and helps reduce cholesterol, a goal for smokers who are at a greater risk for heart disease and stroke.

• Although a serving of shrimp contains 173 milligrams of cholesterol, the damage is offset by its low level of saturated fat: only .2 grams, or 1 gram total fat in a 3-ounce serving.

• Calorie for calorie, protein gives a greater sense of fullness than an equal amount of carbohydrate, so eating fish should allow you to eat fewer calories and feel full longer.

CHICKEN JAMBALAYA
SERVES 5

*J*his slightly spicy, very flavorful version of a Creole favorite contains no added fat. Low-fat smoked sausage and lots of herbs and spices really boost the taste, so you'll never miss the fat-laden original flavor.

1 pound boneless, skinless chicken breasts, cubed

½ pound low-fat fully cooked Polish kielbasa or other smoked sausage, sliced

4 cloves garlic, finely chopped

2 medium onions, chopped

1 green bell pepper, seeded and chopped

1 cup uncooked long grain white rice

1 bay leaf

1 teaspoon Worcestershire sauce

1 teaspoon dried thyme

½ teaspoon cayenne pepper

¼ teaspoon paprika

6 cups low-fat, low-sodium chicken broth

Salt and black pepper to taste

1. Evenly spray a large, heavy saucepan with vegetable oil spray, and place it over high heat. Add the chicken and sausage and sauté for about 5 minutes, stirring occasionally, or until the chicken is golden brown.
2. Reduce the heat to medium. Add the garlic, onions, and bell pepper and sauté for about 4 minutes, or until the vegetables begin to soften. Add the rice, bay leaf, Worcestershire, thyme, cayenne pepper, and paprika and stir to combine. Increase the heat, stir in the chicken broth, and bring the mixture to a boil.
3. Reduce the heat, cover the pan, and simmer the mixture for 20 to 30 minutes, or until the rice is tender. Remove the bay leaf and serve immediately.

Per Serving (2 cups): calories, 370; fat (g), 5; carbohydrates (g), 46; protein (g), 34; cholesterol (mg), 75; sodium (mg), 600.

HEALTH CHECK
- Each serving has only 5 grams of fat.
- Removing skin from chicken substantially lowers its fat and calorie content.
- A mix of aromatic herbs and spices adds flavor without fat, saving on calories that lead to weight gain.
- Chicken is a good source of vitamin B_6, which is generally lacking in smokers' diets.

CHICKEN PICCATA

SERVES 4

*H*ere's an old favorite that takes just minutes to prepare. Serve it with a green vegetable and rice cooked in chicken broth for a quick, tasty, and satisfying meal.

4 boneless, skinless chicken
 breast halves (about 1 pound)
Salt and black pepper to taste
1 tablespoon olive oil
2 tablespoons dry white wine or
 vermouth

¼ cup low-fat, low-sodium
 chicken broth or water
2 tablespoons fresh lemon juice
2 tablespoons capers, rinsed
 and drained

1. Season both sides of the chicken breasts with salt and pepper. In a large nonstick skillet, heat the olive oil over medium-high heat. Add the chicken breasts and cook for about 4 minutes on each side, or until firm, golden brown, and cooked through. Transfer the cooked chicken to a platter and tent with foil while making the pan sauce.

2. Increase the heat to high and add the wine to the pan, stirring with a wooden spoon to scrape the flavorful bits from the bottom of the pan. Add the broth and bring to a boil. Cook, stirring, for about 2 minutes, or until the liquid is reduced by half.

3. Add the lemon juice and capers, bring back to a boil, and remove from the heat. Divide the chicken among plates, spoon a little sauce and capers over each portion, and serve immediately.

Per Serving: calories, 160; fat (g), 5; carbohydrates (g), less than 1 g; protein (g), 26; cholesterol (mg), 66; sodium (mg), 300.

HEALTH CHECK
• This recipe calls for little oil, keeping calories low while still providing enough fat for flavor and satisfaction.
• Each serving has only 5 grams of fat.
• Removing skin from chicken substantially lowers its fat and calorie content.
• Chicken is a good source of vitamin B_6, which is generally lacking in smokers' diets.

CHICKEN "POT ROAST"

SERVES 4

*T*his one-pot dish is great for company because it can be prepared in advance. Removing the skin just before eating reduces the amount of fat.

1 tablespoon olive oil

Salt and black pepper to taste

Juice of ½ a lemon

1 teaspoon dried rosemary

3 cloves garlic, finely chopped

1 whole roasting chicken (about 3 pounds), rinsed and patted

dry (discard the giblets or save for another use)

4 carrots, thickly sliced

4 medium red or white new potatoes, halved

2 large onions, thickly sliced

1. Preheat the oven to 375°F. In a small bowl, combine the olive oil, salt, pepper, lemon juice, rosemary, and garlic, and mash together with the back of a spoon. Rub this mixture evenly over the surface of the chicken.

2. Scatter the carrots, potatoes, and onions over the bottom of a medium roasting pan. Place the chicken breast side up on the vegetables and roast for about 1 hour, or until the skin is crisp, the drumstick moves easily, and the thigh meat reaches 180°F on an instant-read meat thermometer. (The juices should run clear when the thigh is pierced with a knife.) Check the chicken toward the end of roasting and if the vegetables seem in danger of scorching, add a little water to the pan. Let the chicken stand for about 10 minutes before carving. Remove the skin before eating.

Per Serving: calories, 335; fat (g), 7; carbohydrates (g), 41; protein (g), 29; cholesterol (mg), 8; sodium (mg), 120.

HEALTH CHECK

• This dish calls for olive oil, which is primarily a monounsaturated fat and helps to reduce cholesterol, a goal for smokers who are at a greater risk for heart disease and stroke.

• A mix of aromatic herbs adds flavor without fat.

• Chicken is a good source of vitamin B_6, which is generally lacking in smokers' diets.

CHICKEN WITH PEAS

SERVES 4

*A*s a child, one of my favorite foods was a simple chicken dish with a side of peas. This recipe combines both elements in a no-fuss one-pan meal.

1 tablespoon olive oil	⅓ cup dry white wine or
4 boneless, skinless chicken	vermouth
breast halves (about 1 pound)	1 teaspoon dried thyme
Salt and black pepper to taste	2 cups thawed frozen or fresh
1 cup plus 2 tablespoons low-	peas
fat, low-sodium chicken broth	1 tablespoon cornstarch

1. In a large, heavy, nonstick skillet, heat the olive oil over medium-high heat. Season both sides of the chicken breasts with salt and pepper and add to the skillet. Cook for about 3 minutes on each side, or until the chicken is almost firm and golden brown. If the chicken seems in danger of scorching at any time, add a teaspoon of water or broth to the pan.
2. Add 1 cup of the chicken broth, the white wine, and thyme to the skillet. Bring the liquid to a boil and add the peas. Reduce the heat to medium-low, cover the pan, and simmer for about 10 minutes, or until the chicken is cooked through.
3. With a slotted spoon, transfer the chicken and peas to warmed dinner plates. In a small bowl, mix together the cornstarch and the remaining 2 tablespoons of broth, then whisk the mixture into the simmering sauce and cook for about 1 minute, stirring constantly, or until the sauce starts to thicken.
4. Taste for seasoning and add salt and pepper if necessary. Spoon the sauce over the chicken and peas and serve.

Per Serving: calories, 240; fat (g), 6; carbohydrates (g), 12; protein (g), 31; cholesterol (mg), 66; sodium (mg), 330.

HEALTH CHECK
• Chicken is a good source of vitamin B_6, which is generally lacking in smokers' diets.
• Wine and broth increase the moisture in this dish, so less fat is needed.
• Peas provide both fiber and the carbohydrate that increases serotonin in the brain, giving a calming effect.

CHILI-RUBBED BARBECUED CHICKEN

SERVES 4

The dry rub is one of my favorite low-fat, high-flavor cooking tricks. It takes the place of a liquid marinade, and is made with spices and no fat or oil. Try it first as described here with chicken, and then with fish, pork, or beef.

CHILI RUB
2 tablespoons mild chili powder, or to taste
1 tablespoon (firmly packed) light or dark brown sugar
⅛ teaspoon cayenne pepper
4 boneless, skinless chicken breast halves (about 1 pound)
½ cup bottled fat-free hickory barbecue sauce

1. To make the chili rub: In a small bowl, combine the chili powder, brown sugar, and cayenne and toss together.

2. Arrange the chicken breasts in a single layer on a baking sheet. Sprinkle about ¼ teaspoon of the chili rub generously on one side of each breast and rub it lightly into the flesh. Turn over and repeat on the other side. Cover with plastic wrap and let stand at room temperature for 1 hour.

3. Prepare the grill (medium-high heat) or preheat the broiler. If using a grill, be sure to oil the rack so the chicken won't stick. If grilling, place the chicken on the grill rack away from the direct heat, brush generously with the barbecue sauce, and cover the grill. If broiling, place the chicken on the broiler pan and brush generously with the barbecue sauce.

4. Cook the chicken for 15 to 20 minutes, turning every 5 minutes, or until it is cooked through and no trace of pink remains. Baste once or twice during the cooking time with barbecue sauce. (If the sauce seems in danger of scorching during broiling, move the pan farther from the heat.) Serve hot, passing any remaining barbecue sauce separately.

Per Serving: calories, 170; fat (g), 2.5; carbohydrates (g), 8; protein (g), 28; cholesterol (mg), 66; sodium (mg), 370.

HEALTH CHECK
- A mix of aromatic spices adds flavor without fat.
- Removing the skin from chicken substantially lowers its fat and calorie content.
- Chicken is a good source of vitamin B_6, which is generally lacking in smokers' diets.

GRILLED CHICKEN BREASTS WITH BEER

SERVES 4

*H*ere's an oil-free marinade that adds virtually no extra calories but lots of flavor. You can also marinate chicken in lime juice, all by itself. In the winter when it's not practical to use my outdoor barbecue, I like to cook chicken in a ridged nonstick grill pan, which leaves lovely grill-like marks.

¼ cup dark Mexican beer, such as Negro Modelo

¼ cup fresh lime juice

1 tablespoon Tabasco sauce

4 boneless, skinless chicken breast halves (about 1 pound)

1 lime, quartered, for serving

1. In a nonreactive bowl large enough to hold the chicken, mix together the beer, lime juice, and Tabasco. Place the chicken breasts in the marinade and turn to coat them evenly. Cover and marinate at room temperature for at least 1 hour, or in the refrigerator for up to 6 hours (the longer the better).

2. When ready to cook, if the chicken breasts are chilled, let them come to room temperature for 20 minutes. Spray a ridged grill pan with vegetable oil spray and preheat to medium-high heat, or prepare the outdoor grill (medium-high heat), oiling the rack so the chicken won't stick. Remove the chicken breasts from the marinade and pat them thoroughly dry with paper towels. Discard the excess marinade.

3. Grill the breasts for about 6 minutes on each side, or a little longer if on the outdoor grill, or until they are firm and cooked through with no trace of pink remaining. Do not overcook, or they will be dry. Let the chicken stand for 5 minutes, then cut each breast into 4 thick slices and serve with a wedge of lime.

Per Serving: calories, 135; fat (g), 1.5; carbohydrates (g), 2; protein (g), 26; cholesterol (mg), 66; sodium (mg), 75.

HEALTH CHECK

- At only 135 calories per serving, this chicken is a good calorie value.
- Removing the skin from chicken substantially lowers its fat and calorie content.
- A flavorful marinade makes extra fat such as oil or butter unnecessary.
- Chicken is a good source of vitamin B_6, which is generally lacking in smokers' diets.

OVEN-FRIED CHICKEN

SERVES 4

*F*ried chicken is a tough dish to duplicate without fat, but this version is a very tasty alternative. Feel free to spice up the bread crumbs with extra dried herbs for even more flavor. Serve with a green vegetable and Baked Garlic Fries (page 248) for a great meal.

4 boneless, skinless chicken
   breast halves (about 1 pound)
Salt and black pepper to taste
1 cup all-purpose flour

½ cup nonfat milk
1 cup Italian-seasoned bread
   crumbs

1. Preheat the oven to 350°F. Season both sides of the chicken liberally with salt and pepper.

2. Coat a large baking dish evenly with olive oil spray. In three separate shallow bowls, place the flour, milk, and bread crumbs. One piece at a time, dip the chicken: first in flour, turning to coat both sides and shaking off the excess. Then dip in milk to moisten, and finally coat with the bread crumbs. Place the chicken in the prepared baking dish.

3. Spray the chicken pieces lightly with olive oil spray and bake for 15 minutes. Turn over carefully and bake for 10 to 15 minutes more, until the chicken is lightly brown and firm, with no trace of pink remaining. Remove from the oven and serve immediately.

Per Serving: calories, 250; fat (g), 3; carbohydrates (g), 24; protein (g), 31; cholesterol (mg), 66; sodium (mg), 371.

HEALTH CHECK
• Chicken is a good source of vitamin B$_6$, which is generally lacking in smokers' diets.
• Vegetable oil spray, especially olive oil spray, is an easy and almost fat- and calorie-free way to enhance texture and flavor.
• Compare this dish at only 3 grams of fat per serving to traditional fried chicken, which can contain as much as 20 grams of fat per serving!

SMOKY CHICKEN KABOBS

SERVES 4

*K*abobs are a real hit when entertaining and great for the cook, too, because they can be made well in advance. When you're ready, just grill them up and serve. If you use wooden skewers, soak them in water for one hour prior to grilling so they don't burn.

⅓ cup fat-free smoky barbecue
   sauce
⅓ cup orange marmalade
2 tablespoons prepared
   horseradish

4 boneless, skinless chicken
   breast halves (about 1
   pound), cut into ¾-inch cubes

1. In a shallow dish, combine the barbecue sauce, marmalade, and horseradish and stir with a fork to blend. Add the chicken and stir to coat thoroughly with the mixture. Cover with plastic wrap and marinate at room temperature for 30 minutes, or in the refrigerator overnight (the longer the tastier).
2. Prepare the grill (medium-high heat) or preheat the broiler. If using a grill, be sure to oil the rack so the kabobs won't stick. Thread the chicken equally onto 4 metal or wooden skewers and grill the kabobs for about 10 minutes, or until the chicken is cooked through and no trace of pink remains, turning every 3 to 4 minutes. Serve immediately.

Per Serving: calories, 210; fat (g), 2; carbohydrates (g), 21; protein (g), 27; cholesterol (mg), 66; sodium (mg), 260.

HEALTH CHECK
- This marinade adds a nice zip for new ex-smokers whose taste buds are finding new pleasure in eating.
- Chicken is a good source of vitamin B_6, which is generally low in smokers' diets.
- This recipe has only 2 grams of fat per serving.

SUNDAY ROAST CHICKEN

SERVES 4 TO 5

My husband likes to roast a chicken at least one day a week, usually on Sunday. Here's his secret to a delicious and easy dinner. The chicken is stuffed with aromatic vegetables and a quartered lemon, and initially cooked breast side down to keep the breast meat moist.

2 medium onions, coarsely
    chopped
5 cloves garlic, peeled
1 lemon, quartered
1 whole roasting chicken (4 to 5
    pounds), rinsed and patted

dry (discard the giblets or
    save for another use)
¼ cup hot sauce, such as
    chipotle or Tabasco sauce

1. Preheat the oven to 450°F. Place the onions, garlic, and lemon inside the cavity of the chicken. Rub the outside of the chicken with the hot sauce.
2. Place the chicken breast side down on a rack in a roasting pan. Roast for 15 minutes, then reduce the heat to 350°F Roast for 30 minutes more. Turn the chicken breast side up and roast for 1 to 1¼ hours more, or until the drumstick moves easily, the thigh meat reaches 180°F on an instant-read meat thermometer, and the juices run clear with no trace of pink remaining.
3. Remove from the oven and tent the roasting pan very loosely with aluminum foil. Let the chicken stand for 15 to 20 minutes before carving. Discard the flavoring ingredients from the cavity and remove the skin before serving.

Per Serving: calories, 160; fat (g), 2; carbohydrates (g), 8; protein (g), 27; cholesterol (mg), 66; sodium (mg), 80.

HEALTH CHECK

• A 3.5-ounce skinless chicken breast contains 4 grams of fat, whereas the same amount of skinless thigh meat contains 9 grams, a difference of 5 grams of fat (or about 33 calories).
• Chicken is a good source of vitamin B_6, which is generally lacking in smokers' diets.
• Removing the skin from chicken after cooking saves about 5 grams of fat, or about 45 calories per portion.

SWEET AND SOUR CHICKEN STIR-FRY

SERVES 4

*T*his light version of a traditional sweet and sour recipe is not just sweet but absolutely delicious as well! It may be exactly what you need to keep your sweet tooth in check. For a change, replace the chicken with lean pork loin.

2 teaspoons olive oil

1 pound boneless, skinless chicken breasts, cut into small strips

1 16-ounce can pineapple chunks in syrup

¼ cup (firmly packed) light brown sugar

2 tablespoons cornstarch

¼ cup cider vinegar

1½ tablespoons low-sodium soy sauce

1 medium green bell pepper, seeded and cut into small strips

1 medium red bell pepper, seeded and cut into small strips

Thinly sliced green onion (scallion) and sesame seeds, for garnish

4 cups hot steamed rice, for serving

1. In a large nonstick skillet, heat the olive oil over medium heat. Add the chicken and cook for about 2 minutes on each side, or until lightly browned. Add ½ cup of water and bring to a boil. Reduce the heat, cover the pan, and simmer for 5 minutes.
2. While the chicken is cooking, drain the pineapple, reserving the syrup. In a small bowl, combine the brown sugar and cornstarch. Whisk in the reserved pineapple syrup, vinegar, and soy sauce until thoroughly combined.
3. After the chicken has cooked for 5 minutes, increase the heat to medium-high and stir in the pineapple syrup mixture. Cook, stirring constantly, for about 1 minute, or until the sauce thickens. Add the bell peppers and cook for 2 to 3 minutes, stirring, until the peppers soften slightly. Add the pineapple chunks and heat through for 1 minute.

4. Remove from the heat, sprinkle with the green onion and sesame seeds, and serve immediately with the hot rice.

Per Serving: calories, 545; fat (g), 4; carbohydrates (g), 92; protein (g), 33; cholesterol (mg), 66; sodium (mg), 480.

HEALTH CHECK
- This recipe has only 4 grams of fat per serving.
- Peppers add a shot of vitamin C, an antioxidant that helps to destroy the process that can create cancer.
- Vinegar adds a nice zip for new ex-smokers whose taste buds are just waking up.

TERIYAKI CHICKEN

SERVES 4

*T*his dish can be made with lean beef, pork, or ahi tuna instead of chicken, if desired. I love to serve this dish accompanied by rice and pineapple chunks. If using wooden skewers, be sure to soak them in water for one hour first so they don't burn on the grill.

MARINADE
1 cup fat-free teriyaki sauce
¼ cup chopped green onions
   (scallions)
1 teaspoon hot pepper sauce

1 pound boneless, skinless
   chicken breasts, cut into 1-
   inch cubes
8 green onions (scallions), roots
   and very dark green ends
   trimmed away

1. To make the marinade: In a large, shallow bowl, combine the teriyaki sauce, chopped green onions, and hot pepper sauce and whisk together. Add the chicken and whole green onions and stir to coat thoroughly with the mixture. Cover with plastic wrap and marinate in the refrigerator for 1 hour.
2. Prepare the grill (medium-high heat) or preheat the broiler. If using a grill, be sure to oil the rack so the chicken won't stick. Alternately, thread the chicken and green onions onto 4 metal or wooden skewers.
3. Grill the skewers for about 5 minutes on each side, or until the chicken is cooked through and firm with no trace of pink remaining. Serve immediately.

Per Serving: calories, 150; fat (g), 1.5; carbohydrates (g), 5; protein (g), 28; cholesterol (mg), 66; sodium (mg), 780.

HEALTH CHECK
• Removing the skin from chicken lowers the fat content by about 5 grams, or 45 calories per portion.
• This recipe uses an easy marinade instead of extra fat for lots of flavor. It's great for new ex-smokers whose taste buds are waking up after quitting.
• This recipe has only 1½ grams of fat per serving.

WEEKDAY CHICKEN IN WINE

SERVES 4

*T*his special but easy-to-fix chicken is excellent served with steamed broccoli or carrots. For a unique twist, try substituting Marsala wine, which has a sweet, sherrylike flavor. The key is to brown the chicken well before adding the wine.

4 skinless, boneless chicken breast halves (about 1 pound)
Salt and black pepper

1 tablespoon olive oil
½ cup dry white wine or low-fat, low-sodium chicken broth

1. Season the chicken liberally with salt and pepper. In a large nonstick skillet, heat the olive oil over medium-high heat. Add the chicken breasts and cook for about 4 minutes on each side, or until deep golden brown.
2. Add the wine, stirring with a wooden spoon to scrape the flavorful bits from the bottom of the pan and incorporate all the juices. Simmer for about 4 minutes, or until the liquid is reduced by half.
3. Serve the chicken immediately, with the sauce spooned on top.

Per Serving: calories, 175; fat (g), 5; carbohydrates (g), 0; protein (g), 26; cholesterol (mg), 66; sodium (mg), 140.

HEALTH CHECK
• A light sauce of natural meat juices and wine replaces the more traditional cream and butter.
• This low-calorie dish has only 175 calories per serving.
• Removing the skin from chicken substantially lowers its fat and calorie content.

BEEF FAJITAS

SERVES 6

*T*his recipe can also be made with skinless chicken breasts, lean pork loin, or a firm white fish, such as halibut or swordfish. Much of the work can be done in advance, and the presentation is very attractive. Serve as is or wrap the filling in warm tortillas, if you like. To heat tortillas, wrap them in foil and place in a 400°F oven until soft and warm, about 5 minutes.

1 tablespoon canola oil

1 pound round steaks, trimmed of all visible fat and cut into ⅛-inch-thick strips

1 medium onion, halved lengthwise and cut into ¼-inch-thick strips

1 green bell pepper, seeded and cut into ¼-inch-thick strips

1 red bell pepper, seeded and cut into ¼-inch-thick strips

¼ teaspoon dried red pepper flakes

1 tablespoon Worcestershire sauce

Salt and black pepper to taste

6 reduced-fat flour tortillas, warmed (optional)

⅓ cup bottled salsa (optional)

1. In a large cast-iron or heavy nonstick skillet, heat the oil over medium-high heat. Add the beef and cook for 2 minutes, stirring once, then reduce the heat to medium. Add the onion, bell peppers, red pepper flakes, and Worcestershire sauce and cook, stirring occasionally, for about 4 minutes more, or until the vegetables are crisp-tender and the beef firm. Add a teaspoon or two of water if necessary to keep the vegetables from scorching. Season to taste with the salt and pepper.

2. Arrange the beef and vegetables on a large, heated serving platter and serve immediately with warm tortillas and salsa, if desired.

Per Serving: calories, 215; fat (g), 10; carbohydrates (g), 7; protein (g), 25; cholesterol (mg), 73; sodium (mg), 160.

HEALTH CHECK

• Beef scores high in muscle-building and energy-promoting protein and iron, essential nutrients for new ex-smokers who are returning to optimum health.

• Fresh vegetables provide fiber, which helps fill us up so we crave less food and eat fewer calories.

• Well-trimmed lean beef saves on calories and fat grams.

CUBAN-STYLE TURKEY IN TORTILLAS

SERVES 4

*T*urkey and raisins? Together? Yes—and this fabulous flavor combination will surprise you both with its ease and its great taste.

1 medium russet potato, peeled and cut into ¾-inch dice	1 medium onion, finely chopped
1 pound extra-lean (99% fat-free) ground turkey	1 medium green bell pepper, seeded and finely chopped
2 cloves garlic, finely chopped	¼ cup raisins
	4 reduced-fat flour tortillas

1. Bring a medium saucepan of lightly salted water to a boil. Add the potato and cook for 8 minutes, or until tender but not falling apart. Drain and set aside.
2. Preheat the oven to 400°F. In a large nonstick skillet, cook the turkey over medium-high heat for about 6 minutes, stirring frequently and breaking it up with a wooden spoon, or until the turkey is no longer pink. Add the garlic, onion, and bell pepper and cook for about 4 minutes, stirring often, or until the pepper is soft. Add the raisins and the cooked potato and cook for about 2 minutes, stirring, or until the mixture is warmed through. Remove from the heat.
3. While the turkey is cooking, wrap the tortillas in foil, place in the oven, and heat for 5 minutes, or until soft and warm.
4. Divide the turkey mixture among the warmed tortillas. Fold the bottom edge of each tortilla up and over the filling, fold over the sides, and roll up. Serve immediately.

Per Serving: calories, 350; fat (g), 2; carbohydrates (g), 53; protein (g), 33; cholesterol (mg), 56; sodium (mg), 380.

HEALTH CHECK
- This recipe has only 2 grams of fat per serving.
- The protein in turkey increases the feeling of fullness, so you eat less and feel full longer.
- Green bell peppers provide a shot of vitamin C, an antioxidant that helps to destroy the process that creates cancer.

LEAN TURKEY CHILI

SERVES 5

*T*his thick, slightly spicy chili is great served with a salad. Make a pot on the weekend and enjoy it for two or three meals. Or, freeze it in individual containers for lunches and/or last-minute dinners. Top with any garnish you like, as long as it's not high-fat cheese.

2 teaspoons canola oil

1 large onion, chopped

1 large green bell pepper, seeded and chopped

2 cloves garlic, minced

1 pound extra-lean (99% fat-free) ground turkey

2 tablespoons all-purpose flour

2 tablespoons chili powder

1 tablespoon dried oregano or sage, crumbled

2 teaspoons ground cumin

½ teaspoon salt

¼ teaspoon cayenne pepper (optional)

2 14½-ounce cans low-sodium diced tomatoes, with their juice

2 15½-ounce cans low-sodium kidney beans, rinsed and drained

Nonfat plain yogurt, fat-free sour cream, chopped red or green onion, or chopped green bell pepper, for garnish (optional)

1. In a large, deep saucepan, heat the oil over medium-high heat. Add the onion, bell pepper, and garlic and cook for about 5 minutes, stirring occasionally, or until the vegetables have softened. If the vegetables are in danger of scorching at any time, add a tablespoon of water and partially cover the pan. Increase the heat to high, add the turkey and cook for about 5 minutes, stirring frequently and breaking it up with a wooden spoon, or until the turkey is no longer pink.

2. Stir in the flour, chili powder, oregano, cumin, salt, and cayenne, if desired. Cook for about 2 minutes, stirring constantly, or until the flour and spices are well incorporated. Add 3 cups water, the tomatoes with their juice, and the beans. Stir well and bring to a boil.

3. Reduce the heat, partially cover the pan, and simmer for 30 minutes, stirring occasionally, or until the chili is slightly thickened and the flavors blended. Serve immediately, topped with your choice of garnish, if desired.

Per Serving (2 cups): calories, 445; fat (g), 8; carbohydrates (g), 55; protein (g), 43; cholesterol (mg), 62; sodium (mg), 460.

HEALTH CHECK

• This recipe has only 8 grams of fat per 2-cup serving; the same amount of chili made with regular ground beef can contain as much as 60 grams—a difference of over 50 grams of fat.

• Lean turkey replaces fatty ground beef, lowering fat and calories.

• A mix of spices adds a lovely zip for new ex-smokers whose taste buds are waking up.

MEATBALLS

MAKES ABOUT 60 MEATBALLS

I serve these highly seasoned little meatballs as an appetizer with a
small drizzle of bottled spaghetti sauce—they're always eaten down to the
last tasty morsel. Try them with pasta or rice as well for a satisfying main
dish. They're high in protein but low in fat, which is a great combination for
taking the edge off hunger.

2 large egg whites

**2 tablespoons dried Italian herb
seasoning**

½ teaspoon celery salt

1 clove garlic, minced

2 tablespoons ketchup

½ teaspoon Worcestershire sauce

**1½ pounds extra-lean ground
turkey or ground beef (not
exceeding 7% fat)**

**2 tablespoons fine dry bread
crumbs**

1 small onion, finely chopped

1. Preheat the oven to 350°F. Spray 2 baking sheets with olive oil spray. In a
large, chilled mixing bowl, whisk together the egg whites, Italian seasoning,
celery salt, garlic, ketchup, and Worcestershire sauce.

2. Add the ground turkey, bread crumbs, and onion and use your hands to
quickly but thoroughly combine the mixture.

3. Form the mixture into 1-inch balls, using a portion scoop if desired. Place
the meatballs on the prepared baking sheets, making sure they do not touch.
(The meatballs can be refrigerated at this point for up to 24 hours.)

4. Spray the tops of the meatballs evenly with olive oil spray and bake, in
batches if necessary, for about 10 minutes, or until firm and slightly golden.
Serve warm.

Per Serving (5 meatballs): calories, 80; fat (g), 1; carbohydrates (g), 3; protein (g), 15;
cholesterol (mg), 28; sodium (mg), 90.

HEALTH CHECK
- This recipe has only 1 gram of fat per serving.
- A mix of aromatic herbs adds flavor without fat, saving calories to avoid weight
gain.
- These little meatballs are high in protein, which keeps hunger at bay longer than
an equal amount of carbohydrate.

MUSTARD-GLAZED PORK CHOPS

SERVES 4

*D*ijon mustard makes an easy marinade for chicken or beef as well as pork, and you'll be surprised at how flavorful the result is. Cooking nicely tones down the heat of mustard. Feel free to substitute any other favorite mustard, with the exception of Chinese mustard.

4 lean pork loin chops, cut ¾-inch thick (about 4 ounces each), trimmed of all visible fat

2 tablespoons Dijon mustard
¼ teaspoon black pepper
1 teaspoon olive oil
1 medium onion, sliced

1. Nick the pork chops slightly around the edges with a sharp knife to prevent curling during cooking. Coat the chops with the mustard and sprinkle with the pepper. Cover with plastic wrap and marinate at room temperature for 30 minutes, or in the refrigerator overnight (the longer the tastier).

2. In a large nonstick skillet, heat the olive oil over medium heat. Add the onion and cook for about 7 minutes, stirring occasionally, or until browned. Push the onion to the side of the pan and add the pork chops. Cook the chops for about 5 minutes on each side, or until no pink remains and the juices run clear. If the chops seem in danger of scorching at any time, add a tablespoon or so of water to the pan. Serve immediately.

Per Serving: calories, 200; fat (g), 8; carbohydrates (g), 6; protein (g), 26; cholesterol (mg), 71; sodium (mg), 270.

HEALTH CHECK

• Calorie for calorie, protein gives a greater sense of fullness than an equal amount of carbohydrate, so eating pork may allow you to eat less food and feel full longer.

• The chemical galanin may be responsible for our fat cravings. The more fat we eat, the more galanin we produce and the more fat we crave. This dish has just enough fat to satisfy the cravings caused by galanin without a calorie overload.

• Carefully trimming visible fat from pork chops helps keep fat and calorie levels down.

OLD-FASHIONED BEEF STEW
SERVES 4

*I*f you need comfort food during your period of quitting smoking, this new version of an old favorite may just do the trick.

1 pound lean beef chuck,
    trimmed of all visible fat, cut
    into 1-inch cubes
2 tablespoons all-purpose flour
2 tablespoons canola oil
2 large onions, thinly sliced
    (about 3 cups)
2 stalks celery, sliced
2 tablespoons tomato paste
2 cups low-sodium, low-fat beef
    broth

2 cups sliced carrots
2 medium russet potatoes,
    peeled and thinly sliced
    (about 2 cups)
1 tablespoon cornstarch or 2
    additional tablespoons all-
    purpose flour
Salt and black pepper to taste

1. Coat the beef with the flour, shaking off any excess. In a large, heavy non-stick saucepan, heat the oil over medium-high heat. Add the beef and cook for about 6 minutes, or until browned on all sides, turning occasionally. Transfer to a plate with a slotted spoon.

2. Add the onions and celery to the saucepan and cook for 6 minutes, stirring frequently. Return the beef to the saucepan and stir in the tomato paste. Add the broth and enough cold water to just cover the ingredients, 1 to 2 cups. Bring the liquid to a boil, then reduce the heat to low. Partially cover the pan and simmer for about 1¼ hours, or until the beef is tender. Skim off any foam from the top of the liquid.

3. Add the carrots and potatoes to the beef mixture and simmer, partially covered, for 15 to 20 minutes, until the vegetables are tender.

4. In a small bowl, mix together the cornstarch and ¼ cup cold water. Stir the mixture into the stew, increase the heat so that the stew comes to a boil, and cook, stirring constantly, for 1 minute, or until slightly thickened. Season to taste with salt and pepper and serve immediately.

Per Serving (2¼ cups): calories, 490; fat (g), 18; carbohydrates (g), 39; protein (g), 46; cholesterol (mg), 114; sodium (mg), 230.

HEALTH CHECK

• Since this dish has 18 grams of fat per serving, you can make sure you stay within your daily fat allowance of roughly 40 to 60 grams per day (see page 276 to calculate your fat goal) by limiting other fat sources at the meal.

• Choosing lean beef and trimming all visible fat saves on fat and calories.

• Beef scores high in protein and iron, nutrients that can help the new ex-smoker get back to optimum health.

PORK CHOPS WITH APPLESAUCE

SERVES 6

*T*he pairing of tender pork and chunky applesauce is an old favorite and a wonderful flavor combination. This is a quick and easy way to enjoy both. Serve the pork chops with seasoned rice and a green salad.

1 tablespoon olive oil
2 tablespoons finely chopped garlic
2 teaspoons ground cumin
½ teaspoon cayenne pepper
½ teaspoon ground cinnamon
6 lean pork loin chops, cut ¾-

inch thick (about 4 ounces each), trimmed of all visible fat
Salt and black pepper to taste
1½ cups bottled natural applesauce

1. Nick the pork chops slightly around the edges with a sharp knife to prevent curling during cooking. In a shallow dish, combine the oil, garlic, cumin, cayenne pepper, and cinnamon. Add the chops and rub the spice mixture thoroughly into both sides. Cover with plastic wrap and marinate at room temperature for 1 hour, or in the refrigerator overnight.
2. Spray a large nonstick skillet with vegetable oil spray and heat over medium-high heat. Season both sides of the chops with salt and pepper, and add to the skillet. Cook the chops for about 5 minutes on each side, or until no pink remains and the juices run clear. Serve immediately with a dollop of applesauce.

Per Serving: calories, 220; fat (g), 9; carbohydrates (g), 10; protein (g), 26; cholesterol (mg), 71; sodium (mg), 80.

HEALTH CHECK

• This dish calls for olive oil, which is primarily a monounsaturated fat and helps reduce cholesterol. This is a goal for smokers, who are at a greater risk for heart disease and stroke.
• A 4-ounce serving of lean pork contains a comparable amount of fat to the dark meat of chicken.

CHAPTER 16
Pasta and Pizza

Over the last decade, Americans have gladly accepted permission to put carbohydrates on the "good food" list. As a result, pasta and pizza have become trendy foods with gourmet versions of pasta sauces and pizza toppings showing up on restaurant menus everywhere. But now there's bad news: overeating carbohydrate foods, even if prepared without added fat, can be detrimental to those watching their weight.

The good news is that you *can* include pasta and pizza as part of your diet. Go ahead and enjoy them, but don't forget that too many high-carbohydrate foods represent high calories, and high calories mean weight gain. Exercise portion control at all times. Also, to limit calories from pasta, keep any added fat to a bare minimum, and include a salad or a healthy side of broccoli, asparagus, or other low-carb vegetable. When in doubt, have more sauce, less pasta.

Since they are fairly bulky foods, both pasta and pizza contribute to the feeling of fullness, which can help the new ex-smoker who is experiencing cravings. In addition, the carbohydrates in pasta and pizza raise the level of serotonin in the blood, thus pacifying the urge for nicotine.

Try one of the following recipes, like the Fresh Tomato Pasta Toss (page 232), when your craving center signals a deep, urgent hunger! You'll quickly be satisfied, and stay satisfied for hours.

BARBECUED CHICKEN PIZZA

MAKES 8 SLICES, SERVES 2 OR 3

*A*ccording to one of the top national pizza chains, California Pizza Kitchen, barbecued chicken pizza is the most popular pizza. A homemade version is even better, because you can tailor the ingredients to your liking and know you're getting a low-fat pie. Bottled barbecue sauces are often fat-free, but check the label to be sure. Kraft Honey-Hickory barbecue sauce is my favorite. For the crust, use a package of pizza dough from the supermarket refrigerator case or frozen bread dough, fully thawed.

1 teaspoon olive oil

1 small red onion, chopped

1 clove garlic, minced

Salt and black pepper to taste

¾ pound boneless, skinless
  chicken breast tenders

½ cup fat-free hickory barbecue
  sauce

Cornmeal and all-purpose flour,
  for dusting

8 ounces pizza or bread dough,
  at room temperature

½ cup grated Parmesan cheese

1 tablespoon finely chopped
  fresh cilantro

1. In a medium nonstick skillet, heat the olive oil over medium heat. Add the onion and garlic and cook for 5 minutes, stirring occasionally, or until just starting to brown. Season with salt and pepper. Add 1 tablespoon of water and cook for 1 to 2 minutes more, or until the onion is wilted, stirring often. Transfer the mixture to a bowl and return the skillet to the heat.

2. Add ¼ cup of water to the skillet and cook over medium-high heat, scraping all the flavorful bits from the bottom of the pan, until the liquid is reduced by half. Add the chicken and cook for about 5 minutes, or until lightly browned, turning occasionally.

3. Stir in ¼ cup of the barbecue sauce and cook for about 5 minutes more, regulating the heat so the mixture does not scorch, or until the chicken is cooked through with no trace of pink remaining. Remove from the heat.

4. Preheat the oven to 450°F. Spray a baking sheet generously with vegetable oil spray and dust it lightly with cornmeal. On a lightly floured surface, roll out the pizza dough to a large circle or rectangle that will fit on the baking sheet. Transfer the dough to the prepared baking sheet and spread the

remaining ¼ cup barbecue sauce evenly over, leaving a ½-inch border. Scatter the onion mixture evenly over the sauce, then top with the chicken, cheese, and cilantro.

5. Bake for 20 to 25 minutes, or until the topping is bubbling and the crust is golden brown. Serve immediately.

Per Slice: calories, 170; fat (g), 4; carbohydrates (g), 17; protein (g), 16; cholesterol (mg), 30; sodium (mg), 445.

HEALTH CHECK
• Removing the skin from chicken substantially lowers its fat and calorie content.
• Eating low-fat versions of your favorite foods helps you avoid that feeling of deprivation that can lead to diet failure.
• The flavorful barbecue sauce adds moisture to this pizza so you can use less cheese, thus significantly lowering fat and calories.

CHICKEN PARMESAN WITH PASTA

SERVES 4

*A*lthough most gourmet cooks shun bottled spaghetti sauce, most admit that it comes in pretty handy for a last-minute supper. By doctoring up the bottled sauce with onion, celery, wine, and Parmesan, you'll create a delicious version that tastes wonderful served over chicken and pasta.

2 teaspoons olive oil

2 stalks celery, chopped

1 medium onion, chopped

4 boneless, skinless chicken
   breast halves (about 1 pound)

Salt and black pepper to taste

1 cup bottled spaghetti sauce

½ cup dry red or white wine

8 ounces dried spaghetti or your
   favorite noodles

¼ cup grated Parmesan cheese

1. In a large, heavy skillet, heat the olive oil over medium heat. Add the celery and onion and cook for 5 minutes, or until tender, stirring occasionally.
2. Season both sides of the chicken breasts with salt and pepper. Push the vegetables to the side of the skillet and add the chicken. Cook the chicken for about 5 minutes on each side, or until nicely browned.
3. Add the spaghetti sauce and wine and stir to blend. Regulate the heat so the sauce is simmering and cook for about 10 minutes more, or until the chicken is cooked through, turning the chicken once.
4. While the chicken and sauce are cooking, bring a large pot of lightly salted water to a boil and add the spaghetti. Cook until tender according to the package directions.
5. Drain the pasta well and mound onto heated plates. Spoon the chicken and sauce over the pasta, sprinkle with the Parmesan, and serve immediately.

Per Serving: calories, 480; fat (g), 9; carbohydrates (g), 55; protein (g), 38; cholesterol (mg), 71; sodium (mg), 540.

HEALTH CHECK

• Olive oil is primarily a monounsaturated fat, which helps reduce cholesterol.
• The protein in chicken contributes to a feeling of fullness, so you are less likely to overeat the high-carbohydrate pasta.
• The starchy carbohydrates in the pasta will help raise the level of serotonin in the brain and thus calm you down.

FRESH TOMATO PASTA TOSS
SERVES 4

*H*ere's my all-time favorite pasta dish. Since it calls for only fresh ingredients that are minimally cooked, it tastes clean, fresh, and very Italian. You'll find it listed on almost every menu in authentic Italian restaurants, usually as pasta *pomodoro* or spaghetti *alla checca.* I often order an appetizer portion as my entrée.

8 ounces dried spaghettini or
   your favorite noodles
1 tablespoon olive oil
1 medium onion, thinly sliced
3 cloves garlic, thinly sliced

3 ripe plum tomatoes, seeded
   and cut into ¼-inch dice
¼ cup finely chopped fresh basil
   or parsley
Salt and black pepper to taste

1. Bring a large pot of lightly salted water to a boil. Add the pasta and cook until tender according to the package directions.
2. While the pasta is cooking, in a large nonstick skillet, heat the olive oil over medium heat. Add the onion and garlic and cook, stirring occasionally, for about 4 minutes, or until softened.
3. Add the tomatoes to the skillet and cook for about 3 minutes, or until they just start to break down. Add the basil and stir to combine. Season with the salt and pepper.
4. Drain the pasta well and divide it among heated plates. Spoon the sauce over the pasta and serve immediately.

Per Serving: calories, 270; fat (g), 5; carbohydrates (g), 49; protein (g), 8; cholesterol (mg), 0; sodium (mg), 10.

HEALTH CHECK
• Fresh basil adds flavor without fat.
• This recipe calls for olive oil, which is primarily a monounsaturated fat and helps reduce cholesterol. This a worthy goal for smokers, who are at a greater risk for heart disease and stroke.
• Fresh tomatoes add a boost of vitamin C, which is often lacking in smokers' diets.

PASTA WITH PESTO

SERVES 4

*T*rue Italian pesto is made with a mortar and pestle, but a food processor makes this a quick and easy recipe. Pesto freezes well—pack small portions in Ziploc plastic bags and use it anytime to add to pizza toppings, rice, or vegetables. Only a little of this pungent sauce is needed to give a serving of pasta a fresh, clean flavor.

1 cup (packed) fresh basil leaves	¾ teaspoon salt
2 tablespoons pine nuts	3 tablespoons olive oil
2 large garlic cloves, chopped	8 ounces dried pasta of your choice

1. In a food processor, combine the basil, pine nuts, garlic, salt, and half the olive oil. Pulse on and off, scraping down the sides of the bowl as necessary, until the mixture is almost smooth. With the machine running, gradually pour in the remaining olive oil and process until smooth. If the pesto seems dry, mix in a teaspoon or two of water.

2. Bring a large pot of lightly salted water to a boil. Add the pasta and cook according to the package directions. Drain well and transfer to a heated serving bowl.

3. Immediately drizzle the pesto over the pasta and toss thoroughly together. Serve immediately.

Per Serving: calories, 240; fat (g), 14; carbohydrates (g), 44; protein (g), 10; cholesterol (mg), 0; sodium (mg), 400.

HEALTH CHECK

• The chemical galanin may be responsible for our fat cravings. The more fat we eat, the more galanin we secrete and the more fat we crave. This dish has just enough fat to satisfy without a calorie overload.

• When you crave a high-carbohydrate food, your body may need serotonin. Starchy pasta will help raise the serotonin level in your brain and calm you down.

• This recipe calls for olive oil, which is primarily a monounsaturated fat and helps reduce cholesterol, a goal for smokers who are at a greater risk for heart disease and stroke.

PIZZA MARGARITA

SERVES 8

*M*ost of my clients tell me they eat pizza once every week or two, and even more frequently if teenagers are part of the family. By making your own, you eliminate at least half the fat of a store-bought version because there's less oil and less cheese. You can make your own pizza dough; buy Pillsbury's pizza crust in the supermarket refrigerator case, or use frozen bread dough. Some Italian delis and pizzerias sell frozen pizza dough, which is the tastiest option. Just make sure you allow enough time to thaw it at room temperature; it can't be hurried. This is a classic recipe that you'll find in virtually every restaurant in Italy that offers pizza.

Cornmeal or all-purpose flour, for dusting

8 ounces pizza or bread dough, at room temperature

1 tablespoon olive oil

1½ cups shredded part-skim mozzarella cheese (6 ounces)

4 to 5 medium plum tomatoes, thinly sliced

4 cloves garlic, finely chopped

10 fresh basil leaves, finely chopped

1. Preheat the oven to 400°F. Spray a large baking sheet with vegetable oil spray and dust with cornmeal. On a lightly floured surface, roll out the dough into a large circle or rectangle that will fit on the baking sheet. (Let it rest for a few minutes, covered with a kitchen towel, if it resists stretching out to the desired size.) Resume stretching. You may also divide the dough into 4 balls and shape each one into an individual round, pressing outward with your fingertips.

2. Brush the dough with the olive oil, then sprinkle with half the cheese. Arrange the tomato slices over the cheese and scatter over the garlic, basil, and remaining cheese.

3. Bake the large pizza for 20 to 25 minutes and the small ones for 15 to 20 minutes, or until the topping is bubbly and the crust is golden and crisp. Serve immediately.

Per Serving: calories, 155; fat (g), 6; carbohydrates (g), 16; protein (g), 9; cholesterol (mg), 11; sodium (mg), 260.

HEALTH CHECK
- Garlic and basil provide lots of flavor without adding fat or calories to speak of.
- Using part-skim mozzarella rather than whole-milk cheese reduces the fat content considerably.
- Fresh vegetables give a boost of fiber that contributes to a feeling of fullness, which should last throughout the evening and prevent the return of cravings.

SPINACH AND ZUCCHINI LASAGNA

SERVES 12

$\mathcal{T}$his do-ahead dish is great for weekend cooks or those who want to pull out an impressive dish for unexpected guests. It can be made a day or two in advance and refrigerated, or frozen for up to 6 weeks. If baking from frozen, bake, covered with foil, for 1 hour and 15 minutes, then uncover and proceed as directed. Substitute ground turkey or lean ground beef for the spinach, if you like.

1 tablespoon olive oil

1 large onion, chopped

3 cloves garlic, finely chopped

2 cups (packed) chopped fresh spinach, or thawed frozen chopped, drained well

2 cups grated zucchini

1 15-ounce tub part-skim ricotta cheese

1 large egg, lightly beaten

½ teaspoon salt

¼ teaspoon black pepper

6 cups bottled tomato and basil spaghetti sauce

8 ounces "no-cook" lasagna noodles

½ cup shredded part-skim mozzarella cheese (2 ounces)

¼ cup grated Parmesan cheese

1. Preheat the oven to 350°F. In a medium saucepan, heat the olive oil over medium heat. Add the onion and garlic and cook for 4 to 5 minutes, or until softened. Add the spinach and zucchini and cook for 2 minutes, or until the spinach has wilted. Remove from the heat and cool.

2. In a large bowl, combine the ricotta, egg, salt, and pepper and mix well. Stir in the zucchini and spinach mixture.

3. In a 13 × 9 × 2-inch baking pan, spread 2 cups of the spaghetti sauce to cover the bottom. Top with 3 or 4 lasagna noodles, arranging them in a single layer. Carefully spread half of the ricotta-vegetable mixture over the noodles. Cover with another 2 cups of sauce, then the remaining noodles and ricotta mixture. Spoon over the remaining 2 cups of sauce. (At this point, the lasagna can be covered and refrigerated for up to two days or frozen for up to 6 weeks.)

4. Cover the pan with aluminum foil and bake for 35 minutes, or until the sauce begins to bubble. Remove the foil, sprinkle with the cheeses, and bake for 15 minutes more. Remove the lasagna from the oven and let stand for 10 minutes before cutting and serving.

Per Serving: calories, 250; fat (g), 11; carbohydrates (g), 30; protein (g), 12; cholesterol (mg), 33; sodium (mg), 870.

HEALTH CHECK
• Pasta contains carbohydrates that raise the level of serotonin in the blood, which may help to pacify the urge for nicotine.
• Delicious low-fat cheeses replace the full-fat cheeses of a traditional lasagna, saving about 10 grams of fat and nearly 100 calories per serving.

CHAPTER 17
Sandwiches
and Wraps

Sandwiches make an ideal lunch or light dinner. But when you buy one from a restaurant or deli, you're likely to get too much bread and meat, not to mention mayonnaise or "special sauce." It's helpful to be specific when you order (hold the mayo, limit the filling, no cheese). And if the sandwich is huge, eat half and save the remainder for the next day's lunch.

When you make your own, however, you'll always "have it your way." The recipes that follow are easy to assemble for a meal at home or a brown bag to go. Each is a great-tasting sandwich combination that fits right into a balanced diet. You'll find some new ideas here to enrich your repertoire, as well as leaner versions of old favorites, including Bagels with Cream Cheese and Salmon (page 239), BBQ Pork Sandwiches (page 240), French Onion Turkey Burgers (page 243), and a standby from my childhood, Sloppy Joes (page 244). For those who like a handheld construction wrapped in a tortilla, try the Easy Ham and Cheese Quesadillas (page 242), Tex-Mex Bean and Cheese Burritos (page 245), or the Veggie Wraps (page 246).

BAGELS WITH CREAM CHEESE AND SALMON

SERVES 4

*L*ox and bagels, an excellent brunch item, never goes out of style. For a gourmet twist, top these tasty sandwiches with the Crunchy Cucumber Slices on page 190. I prefer whipped low-fat cream cheese to the nonfat variety, but take your pick.

4 bagels, halved

6 ounces low-fat whipped cream cheese

8 ounces thinly sliced smoked salmon or lox

Lemon wedges, for serving (optional)

1. Toast the bagels until golden. (If done in batches, keep them warm in a napkin-lined basket.)

2. Spread a thin layer of cream cheese over both sides of each bagel, and then place 1 slice of salmon on 1 side. Serve, accompanied by a wedge of lemon, if desired.

Per Serving: calories, 315; fat (g), 8; carbohydrates (g), 38; protein (g), 20; cholesterol (mg), 26; sodium (mg), 940.

HEALTH CHECK
• Low-fat whipped cream cheese takes the place of regular cream cheese, saving calories and fat, and it also spreads more easily so you use less.
• Bagels are a form of complex carbohydrate that can raise the level of serotonin in the blood and thus help to pacify the urge for nicotine.
• Calorie per calorie, protein gives a greater sense of fullness than an equal amount of carbohydrate, so adding salmon to your bagel may allow you to eat less food and feel full longer.

BBQ PORK SANDWICHES

SERVES 4

*T*his is a delicious and satisfying sandwich with less than a third of the calories of a Big Mac, and lots of that yummy barbecue flavor. The pork mixture will keep for up to four days in the refrigerator.

½ cup fat-free barbecue sauce

¼ cup rice wine vinegar

1 teaspoon chili powder

1 pound boneless pork loin,

trimmed of all visible fat, cut into ½-inch dice

4 whole-wheat hamburger buns, split and toasted

1. In a shallow dish, blend the barbecue sauce, vinegar, and chili powder. Add the pork and toss to coat evenly. Cover and marinate at room temperature for 30 minutes, or in the refrigerator overnight.

2. Heat a large nonstick skillet over medium-high heat until hot. Add the pork and its marinade and cook, tossing occasionally, for about 5 minutes, or until firm. Cover the skillet and reduce the heat to low. Simmer for 5 minutes more.

3. Spoon the pork mixture onto the bun bottoms, cover with the tops, and serve immediately.

Per Serving: calories, 315; fat (g), 9; carbohydrates (g), 27; protein (g), 30; cholesterol (mg), 71; sodium (mg), 590.

HEALTH CHECK
- This recipe has only 9 grams of fat per serving.
- Vinegar and barbecue sauce add rich flavor without fat for new ex-smokers whose taste buds are just reawakening.
- Lean, trimmed pork—which saves on calories and fat—gives a jolt of protein, making you feel full longer.

CHICKEN SALAD SANDWICHES

SERVES 2

*W*henever I cook chicken for dinner, I always prepare enough for chicken salad sandwiches the next day. This simple combination of ingredients really does the trick for a light but luscious sandwich. The chicken salad could also be served on a bed of salad greens. It will keep, covered and chilled, for up to 24 hours.

DRESSING
¼ cup light mayonnaise
1 tablespoon whole-grain mustard
1 teaspoon fresh lemon juice
Salt and black pepper to taste

8 ounces cooked chicken, cut into ½-inch dice (approximately

half the meat from a 3-pound roast chicken, see page 214), or 2 cooked boneless, skinless chicken breast halves, diced
1 stalk celery, cut into ¼-inch dice
¼ medium onion, cut into ¼-inch dice
4 slices whole-wheat bread

1. To make the dressing: In a large bowl, whisk together the mayonnaise, mustard, and lemon juice. If desired, thin with water to a nice coating consistency. Whisk in salt and pepper.
2. Fold the diced chicken, celery, and onion into the dressing until well mixed. Taste for seasoning. Serve on the bread as a sandwich,.

Per Serving: calories, 330; fat (g), 8; carbohydrates (g), 32; protein (g), 32; cholesterol (mg), 76; sodium (mg), 670.

HEALTH CHECK
• Removing the skin from chicken substantially lowers its fat and calorie content.
• Protein increases satiety, so you eat less and feel full longer.
• Light mayonnaise replaces regular mayonnaise, reducing fat by about 5 grams and calories by about 45 per serving.

EASY HAM AND CHEESE QUESADILLAS
SERVES 2

*I*f your newly awakened taste buds are responding well to spicy foods, add a bit of your favorite hot sauce or salsa to these quesadillas. You could also include the Refried Bean Dip from page 169.

2 8-inch reduced-fat flour
tortillas
⅔ cup reduced-fat cheddar
cheese (about 3 ounces)
2 tablespoons drained chopped
canned green chilies

4 ounces lean ham slices,
chopped
⅓ cup bottled chunky salsa
1 tablespoon fat-free sour
cream (optional)

1. Spray a large nonstick skillet with vegetable oil spray and place over medium heat. Add 1 tortilla and sprinkle evenly with half the cheese, leaving a ¼-inch border. Scatter over the chilies and ham, and then add the remaining cheese. Place the remaining tortilla on top and press down gently with the palm of your hand.
2. Heat for 3 to 4 minutes, or until the cheese begins to melt and the bottom tortilla is slightly browned. Press down again to "cement" the tortillas together. Flip the quesadilla carefully and heat for another 3 to 4 minutes, or until the cheese is fully melted and the tortilla is slightly browned.
3. Transfer the quesadilla to a cutting board and cut into 8 wedges with a large knife or pizza cutter. Serve the wedges immediately with the salsa and, if desired, the fat-free sour cream.

Per Serving: calories, 340; fat (g), 12; carbohydrates (g), 29; protein (g), 25; cholesterol (mg), 57; sodium (mg), 1,690.

HEALTH CHECK
• By using low-fat versions of ingredients such as sour cream, tortillas, and cheese instead of their full-fat counterparts, you save about 7 grams of fat per serving.
• Protein from ham, carbohydrates from tortillas, and a little fat from the cheese make this festive dish almost perfect nutritionally.

FRENCH ONION TURKEY BURGERS

SERVES 4

*W*hen I was first married, my husband was in the habit of going out to his favorite greasy burger joint to get his weekend fix. Now I keep healthy burger fixings on hand and he makes his own on Saturday afternoon.

1 pound extra-lean (99% fat-free) ground turkey	2 medium onions, thinly sliced
1 large egg white	4 poppyseed French rolls or rolls of your choice, split
1 clove garlic, finely chopped	1 tablespoon Dijon mustard
½ teaspoon salt	4 leaves firm lettuce, such as iceberg
¼ teaspoon freshly ground black pepper	1 large tomato, sliced

1. In a bowl, combine the ground turkey, egg white, garlic, salt, and pepper. Mix together with your hands until thoroughly combined, then form into 4 equal balls. Flatten the balls with the palms of your hands into patties.

2. Heat a large nonstick skillet over medium-high heat. Place the patties in the pan with the sliced onions scattered around them. Cook the burgers and onions, adding a tablespoon or two of water to prevent scorching if necessary, for 15 to 20 minutes, using a plastic spatula to stir the onions and turn the burgers, or until the burgers are firm and no trace of pink remains in the center.

3. While the burgers are cooking, toast the cut sides of the French rolls in a toaster oven or under the broiler. Spread both sides of each roll thinly with the mustard, and serve each burger on the bottom half. Top with some of the cooked onion, a lettuce leaf, a few tomato slices, and the top of the bun. Serve immediately.

Per Serving: calories, 375; fat (g), 7; carbohydrates (g), 36; protein (g), 41; cholesterol (mg), 77; sodium (mg), 700.

HEALTH CHECK
- This recipe has only 7 grams of fat per serving.
- Lean turkey replaces fatty ground beef, saving over 20 grams of fat and about 200 calories.
- A bit of garlic adds flavor to turkey without fat, saving calories and avoiding weight gain.

SLOPPY JOES

SERVES 6

*I*n the Midwest, where I'm from, this was a regular on school lunch menus, concession stands, and at home on Saturday afternoon. Sloppy Joes are also known—somewhat obscurely—as maid rites, beef treats, and taverns! Whatever the name, my version works beautifully as a low-fat sandwich.

1 pound extra-lean ground beef (not exceeding 7% fat) or turkey

½ cup finely chopped onion

½ cup ketchup

2 teaspoons hot mustard

1 teaspoon Worcestershire sauce

Dash of chili powder (optional)

Salt and black pepper to taste

6 whole-wheat hamburger buns, split

1. Heat a large nonstick skillet over medium-high heat. Add the ground beef and onion and cook for 6 to 8 minutes, breaking the meat up with a wooden spoon, until the meat is no longer pink. Drain off any excess fat and return the skillet to the heat.

2. Add the ketchup, mustard, Worcestershire sauce, and chili powder, if desired. Mix well and cook for 1 to 2 minutes more, until thoroughly combined and heated through.

3. Season with salt and pepper and serve immediately on the hamburger buns.

Per Serving: calories, 365; fat (g), 15; carbohydrates (g), 30; protein (g), 27; cholesterol (mg), 81; sodium (mg), 620.

HEALTH CHECK

• Using extra-lean ground beef instead of regular ground beef saves about 15 grams of fat and 135 calories.

• Beef scores high in muscle-building, energy-promoting protein and iron, important nutrients for those who are trying to return to optimum health after quitting smoking.

• A mix of sweet, hot, and tangy seasonings provides flavor without adding fat.

TEX-MEX BEAN AND CHEESE BURRITOS

SERVES 2

*B*urritos can be a high-fat indulgence when laden with lots of cheese, sour cream, and meat. This lightened version won't wreak havoc on a healthy diet, but it's still very tasty. Try it on a traditional burrito lover and watch the reaction!

2 large reduced-fat flour
  tortillas
1 cup fat-free refried beans
4 tablespoons mild red bottled
  salsa
½ cup shredded red cabbage
4 tablespoons fat-free sour
  cream

¼ cup coarsely chopped fresh
  cilantro
½ cup shredded reduced-fat
  cheddar cheese (2 ounces)
2 green onions (scallions), white
  and light green parts only,
  thinly sliced

1. Preheat the oven to 350°F. Wrap the tortillas in aluminum foil and heat in the oven for about 5 minutes, or until warm and soft. Meanwhile, in a small saucepan, heat the beans over medium-low heat until bubbling.

2. On each warm tortilla, spread ½ cup of the refried beans, 2 tablespoons of the salsa, and ¼ cup of the cabbage. Top each with 2 tablespoons sour cream, half of the cilantro, and ¼ cup of the cheese. Sprinkle over the green onions, roll up tightly, and serve immediately.

Per Serving: calories, 340; fat (g), 9; carbohydrates (g), 47; protein (g), 19; cholesterol (mg), 20; sodium (mg), 1,120.

HEALTH CHECK
• This recipe has only 9 grams of fat per serving.
• By using low-fat versions of tortillas, beans, sour cream, and cheese instead of their full-fat counterparts, you save about 9 grams of fat or 80 calories per serving.

VEGGIE WRAPS
SERVES 2

*T*his recipe is a great way to fit more vegetables into your diet, plus it's easy and tasty.

2 8-inch reduced-fat flour tortillas
½ cup reduced-fat cream cheese
½ medium cucumber, peeled,
   halved lengthwise, seeded,
   and thinly sliced

1 plum tomato, thinly sliced
2 thin slices red onion
Salt and black pepper to taste

On each tortilla, spread ¼ cup of the cream cheese, leaving a ¼-inch border. Divide the cucumber, tomato, and red onion between each, and season generously with salt and pepper. Roll up tightly, cut wrap in half, and serve immediately.

Per Serving: calories, 270; fat (g), 10; carbohydrates (g), 34; protein (g), 10; cholesterol (mg), 30; sodium (mg), 740.

HEALTH CHECK
• Using reduced-fat versions of ingredients such as tortillas and cream cheese saves about 4 grams of fat and 40 calories.
• Fresh vegetables give a boost of fiber with relatively few calories—and fiber gives a feeling of fullness that should last throughout the afternoon.
• Tortillas are a form of complex carbohydrate that can raise the level of serotonin in the blood, which may help to pacify the urge for nicotine.

CHAPTER 18
Side Dishes

For many of us, Mom's square meal was meat, a starch, and a vegetable. If your taste buds are used to plain vegetables with the same old potato or rice, your newly awakened appetite may appreciate a little diversity. Capitalize on the versatility of bland starches; their very plainness suggests that the only limit is your imagination. Try Roasted Rosemary Potatoes (page 255), Potato Pancakes (page 254), or Fried Rice (page 252). Balancing your meal by including plenty of great-tasting vegetables will be easy with dishes like Broccoli with Mock Hollandaise Sauce (page 249), Carrots and Zucchini with Sesame and Soy (page 250), and Sautéed String Beans with Walnuts and Lemon (page 257).

For vegetarians, side dishes with plenty of pizzazz can easily become the main meal. But vegetarians may need to find other ways to fulfill their body's protein requirement. Depending on your vegetarian philosophy, fish, eggs, cheeses, nuts, and grains can add protein to your diet. But beware of over-cheesing foods as a protein ploy. Nuts are high in fat as well, so calculate your daily calorie and fat goals and fit the protein boost into that plan.

BAKED GARLIC FRIES

SERVES 4

*H*ere's a low-fat, garlicky version of the perennial diet-destroyer, French fries. These are easy to prepare and pack so much great flavor that you honestly won't miss the fat. Serve with ketchup, if desired. Cut the potatoes when ready to cook to prevent discoloration.

1 tablespoon olive oil
2 large cloves garlic, finely
   chopped
3 medium russet potatoes

(about 2 pounds), cut into ¼-
   inch-thick matchsticks
½ teaspoon salt, or to taste

1. Preheat the oven to 425°F. Spray a large baking sheet with vegetable oil spray and set aside.
2. In a medium bowl, combine the olive oil and garlic. Add the potatoes and toss to coat well.
3. Spread the potatoes in a single layer on the prepared baking sheet and bake for 40 minutes, or until golden brown, turning the potatoes occasionally with a spatula so they brown evenly. Season with the salt and serve immediately.

Per Serving: calories, 210; fat (g), 3.5; carbohydrates (g), 41; protein (g), 5; cholesterol (mg), 0; sodium (mg), 225.

HEALTH CHECK
• These fries have 3.5 grams of fat per serving, versus 18 grams of fat for regular French fries. That represents a savings of about 150 calories.
• This recipe calls for olive oil, primarily a monounsaturated fat, rather than the saturated fats typically used for frying French fries. Monounsaturated fats help reduce cholesterol, a goal for smokers who are at a greater risk for heart disease and stroke.

BROCCOLI WITH MOCK
HOLLANDAISE SAUCE
SERVES 4

*I*f you can't face plain steamed broccoli, this simple and delicious sauce is sure to bring new life to the nutritious vegetable. Use broccoli stems as well as the florets; the stems will cook more evenly if you peel them before cooking. Broccoli is a great source of fiber and vitamins.

¼ cup light mayonnaise
1 tablespoon fresh lemon juice
Salt and black pepper to taste

1 pound broccoli, florets cut into roughly equal pieces, stems peeled and cut into 2-inch-long matchsticks

1. In a small bowl, combine the mayonnaise, lemon juice, salt, and pepper and whisk until well combined. Set aside.
2. In a large saucepan, bring about 2 inches of lightly salted water to a boil. Place the broccoli in a steamer basket over the boiling water, cover the pan, and steam for about 10 minutes, or until tender. Serve immediately with the hollandaise sauce on the side, or toss gently with the sauce.

Per Serving: calories, 85; fat (g), 5; carbohydrates (g), 7; protein (g), 3; cholesterol (mg), 5; sodium (mg), 210.

HEALTH CHECK
• Broccoli gives a boost of fiber with relatively few calories, a great alternative when you're tempted to reach for a cigarette.
• Delicious low-fat mayonnaise replaces regular mayonnaise and saves about 6 grams of fat and 50 calories per serving.
• Broccoli is a member of the cruciferous family of vegetables, which contain substances that help prevent cancerous tumors from developing.

CARROTS AND ZUCCHINI WITH SESAME AND SOY

SERVES 4

*T*he deceptively simple but quite delicious seasonings of lemon juice, soy sauce, and sesame seeds can be used with any combination of vegetables. Blanching denser vegetables before stir-frying decreases the amount of oil needed.

½ pound carrots, cut into ¼-inch-thick matchsticks

1 tablespoon olive oil

½ pound zucchini, cut into ¼-inch-thick matchsticks

1 tablespoon low-sodium soy sauce

1 tablespoon fresh lemon juice

Salt and black pepper to taste

1 teaspoon sesame seeds, toasted (optional)

1. Bring a large pot of lightly salted water to a boil. Add the carrots and cook for 2 minutes, then drain and immediately rinse under cold running water to stop the cooking. Set aside.

2. In a large nonstick or cast-iron skillet, heat the olive oil over medium-high heat. Add the zucchini, carrots, soy sauce, and lemon juice and cook for 2 minutes, tossing constantly. Remove from the heat. Season with the salt and pepper, sprinkle with the sesame seeds, if desired, and serve.

Per Serving: calories, 70; fat (g), 4; carbohydrates (g), 8; protein (g), 2; cholesterol (mg), 0; sodium (mg), 150.

HEALTH CHECK

• This recipe has only 70 calories per serving.

• Fresh vegetables are packed with fiber, which fills you up quickly so you eat less food.

• Soy sauce and lemon juice provide a nice zip for new ex-smokers whose taste buds are waking up.

DRY-ROASTED GREEN BEANS WITH GARLIC AND SOY SAUCE

SERVES 4

*I*f you like French fries, you'll love the unique flavor of these crispy treats that contain a fraction of the fat. You may want to adjust the roasting time depending on how crunchy you like your beans. The amount of garlic can also be adjusted according to taste. Serve as a snack, or as an excellent accompaniment to a salad or sandwich.

4 cloves garlic, halved	Black pepper to taste
2 tablespoons low-sodium soy sauce	1 pound thin green beans, trimmed
1 tablespoon olive oil	2 teaspoons fresh lemon juice

1. Preheat the oven to 400°F. Spray a roasting pan evenly with olive oil spray and place it in the oven to heat up.
2. In a large bowl, combine the garlic, soy sauce, olive oil, and black pepper. Add the green beans and toss until evenly coated with the mixture.
3. When the oven and the roasting pan are very hot, transfer the beans to the hot pan. Roast for about 40 minutes, tossing occasionally, or until the beans are very crunchy. Serve hot.

Per Serving: calories, 75; fat (g), 4; carbohydrates (g), 10; protein (g), 3; cholesterol (mg), 0; sodium (mg), 520.

HEALTH CHECK
- These beans contain only 75 calories per serving.
- This recipe calls for very little oil, keeping calories low while still providing enough fat for flavor and satisfaction.
- The fiber in green beans will fill you up quickly and keep you feeling full longer.

FRIED RICE

SERVES 4

*T*his dish is a great way to use up any odd vegetables in the refrigerator, not to mention that leftover rice from last night's dinner. If leftover rice is not available, simmer ½ cup rice in 1¼ cups salted water for 15 minutes, cover, let stand for 5 minutes, and fluff with a fork. For a shot of protein, add a lightly beaten egg with the rice when adding the soy sauce.

1 teaspoon sesame oil
1 medium zucchini, cut into ½-inch dice
1 cup chopped mushrooms
1 stalk celery, cut into ½-inch dice

1 cup cooked white or brown rice
1 teaspoon low-sodium soy sauce

1. In a large nonstick skillet, heat the sesame oil over medium heat. Add the zucchini, mushrooms, and celery and cook for 2 to 3 minutes, until the vegetables just start to soften.
2. Add the rice and soy sauce and toss with the vegetables until just warmed through and well combined. Serve immediately.

Per Serving: calories, 75; fat (g), 1.5; carbohydrates (g), 14; protein (g), 2; cholesterol (mg), 0; sodium (mg), 55.

HEALTH CHECK
• This recipe has just 75 calories per serving.
• Vegetables like zucchini contain fiber, which fills us up quickly so we eat less food.
• When you crave a high-carbohydrate food, your body may need the serotonin boost that it used to receive from nicotine. The starch in rice helps raise the serotonin level in your brain and thus calm you down.

ITALIAN-STYLE SPAGHETTI SQUASH

SERVES 4

*S*paghetti squash is definitely a fun food. When you cut it open, the inside comes out in pastalike strands, and the lovely flavor makes a heavy sauce unnecessary. The traditional Italian garnish of parsley, lemon zest, garlic, and black pepper known as *gremolata* packs a big wallop of flavor without fat.

1 small spaghetti squash (about 2 pounds), halved lengthwise and seeded

1 tablespoon olive oil

2 small cloves garlic, finely chopped

2 tablespoons finely chopped fresh parsley

2 teaspoons finely chopped lemon zest

Salt and coarsely ground black pepper to taste

1. In a large saucepan, bring about 2 inches of lightly salted water to a boil. Place the squash in a steamer basket over the boiling water, cover the pan, and steam for about 20 minutes, or until tender. Set aside until cool enough to handle.
2. Using a fork, scoop out the squash into a colander and drain off the excess water.
3. In a large nonstick skillet, heat the olive oil over medium heat. Add the garlic and cook for 2 minutes, stirring frequently. Add the squash and cook for 5 minutes, or until slightly golden, stirring often.
4. Remove the squash mixture from the heat and add the parsley, lemon zest, salt, and pepper. Toss together quickly and serve immediately.

Per Serving: calories, 100; fat (g), 4; carbohydrates (g), 16; protein (g), 2; cholesterol (mg), 35; sodium (mg), 110.

HEALTH CHECK
- This recipe has only 4 grams of fat per serving.
- A mix of aromatic herbs adds flavor without fat, saving calories to avoid weight gain.
- Fresh vegetables give a boost of fiber with relatively few calories, keeping you feeling full longer.

POTATO PANCAKES

SERVES 4

*T*hese pancakes are reminiscent of old-fashioned hash brown potatoes. Here, however, I use egg and flour to hold them together instead of butter. By using a nonstick pan and a small amount of oil, they get deliciously brown and crispy. I usually make extra pancakes and reheat them in the microwave the next day.

2 large or 4 medium russet
   potatoes (about 1½ pounds),
   peeled
1 small onion
1 large egg
Salt and black pepper to taste

1 tablespoon all-purpose flour
1 tablespoon canola oil
Fat-free sour cream, chopped
   green onions (scallions), or
   applesauce, for serving

1. Preheat the oven to 200°F. Using a box grater or food processor, coarsely grate the potatoes and onion. Combine them in a large colander and press to drain off the excess moisture. Set aside.
2. In a medium bowl, beat together the egg, salt, and pepper. Stir in the flour, then the grated potatoes and onion until thoroughly mixed.
3. In a large nonstick skillet, heat the oil over medium heat. For each pancake, place about 2 heaping tablespoons of the potato mixture in the pan and press down to form a flat patty. Cook for 4 to 5 minutes on each side, or until golden brown.
4. Transfer to paper towels to blot off excess oil. Place on a paper towel–lined baking sheet and keep warm in the oven while cooking the remainder. Serve immediately with fat-free sour cream, green onions, or applesauce.

Per Serving: calories, 205; fat (g), 5; carbohydrates (g), 36; protein (g), 6; cholesterol (mg), 53; sodium (mg), 95.

HEALTH CHECK
• This recipe has only 5 grams of fat per serving.
• When you crave a high-carbohydrate food, your brain may be in need of the serotonin that was previously boosted by nicotine. The starch in potatoes will help raise the serotonin level in your brain and calm you down.
• Browned potatoes provide a crunch that soothes the need for oral gratification.

ROASTED ROSEMARY POTATOES
SERVES 4

*H*ere's an old favorite that goes nicely with roasted meats, fish, or chicken.

1 tablespoon olive oil

2 tablespoons chopped fresh rosemary, or 2 teaspoons dried, crumbled

3 large russet potatoes (about 2 pounds), thinly sliced into rounds

Salt and black pepper to taste

1. Preheat the oven to 425°F. Lightly coat a large baking sheet with vegetable oil spray. In a medium bowl, combine the oil and rosemary. Add the sliced potatoes and toss together to coat evenly.

2. Spread the potatoes evenly on the prepared baking sheet and sprinkle with the salt and pepper. Roast for 40 to 45 minutes, turning once with a spatula, until golden brown and tender. Serve immediately.

Per Serving: calories, 210; fat (g), 4; carbohydrates (g), 41; protein (g), 5; cholesterol (mg), 0; sodium (mg), 280.

HEALTH CHECK
- Each serving has only 4 grams of fat.
- Rosemary provides lots of flavor without adding fat.
- This dish calls for olive oil, which is primarily a monounsaturated fat and helps reduce cholesterol, a goal for smokers who are at a greater risk for heart disease and stroke.

STIR-FRIED SNOW PEAS WITH GARLIC AND GINGER

SERVES 4

*T*his elegant dish is a wonderful accompaniment to grilled fish or chicken, and the combination of colorful vegetables makes an attractive presentation.

1 teaspoon canola oil

½ teaspoon sesame oil

½ pound snow peas, trimmed (about 2 cups)

½ medium red bell pepper, seeded and cut into ¼-inch-wide strips

6 large cloves garlic, thinly sliced

1 tablespoon low-sodium soy sauce

1 teaspoon minced fresh ginger

1. In a large, heavy, nonstick skillet, heat the canola and sesame oils over medium-high heat. Add the snow peas, cover the pan, and cook for 2 minutes, shaking the pan vigorously once or twice during the cooking time.
2. Add the red pepper, garlic, soy sauce, and ginger and stir-fry for about 3 minutes, or until the snow peas are crisp-tender. Serve immediately.

Per Serving: calories, 105; fat (g), 4; carbohydrates (g), 14; protein (g), 5; cholesterol (mg), 0; sodium (mg), 260.

HEALTH CHECK

• Aromatic fresh ginger adds flavor without fat, saving calories to avoid weight gain.

• Fresh vegetables give a boost of fiber with relatively few calories, keeping you feeling full longer.

• Red bell pepper provides a shot of vitamin C, which is generally lacking in smokers' diets. Vitamin C is an antioxidant that may help to destroy the process that forms cancer cells.

SAUTÉED GREEN BEANS WITH WALNUTS AND LEMON

SERVES 2

*T*his recipe came to me from the Grange Hall restaurant in New York City's Greenwich Village. The walnuts give the dish a nice crunch and the lemon adds a bit of a kick. Be sure not to overcook the beans.

2 cups green beans, trimmed

1 teaspoon olive oil

2 tablespoons coarsely chopped walnuts

1 tablespoon grated lemon zest

1 tablespoon fresh lemon juice

Salt and black pepper to taste

Lemon wedges, for serving

1. Bring a large pot of lightly salted water to a boil. Meanwhile, fill a large bowl with ice and cold water. Add the beans to the boiling water and cook for 1 minute. Drain and transfer immediately to the ice water. Let stand in the ice water, then drain and set aside on paper towels.

2. In a large nonstick skillet, heat the olive oil over medium heat. Add the walnuts and lemon zest and cook for about 2 minutes, or until the walnuts begin to brown, stirring constantly. Add the beans and cook for 2 to 3 minutes, until the beans are warmed through.

3. Add the lemon juice, salt, and pepper and toss together gently. Serve immediately, with the lemon wedges on the side.

Per Serving: calories, 105; fat (g), 7; carbohydrates (g), 11; protein (g), 3; cholesterol (mg), 0; sodium (mg), 140.

HEALTH CHECK
• The fat in nuts is mostly monounsaturated and helps reduce cholesterol, a goal for smokers who are at a greater risk for heart disease and stroke.
• Crisp vegetables provide a crunch that soothes the need for oral gratification.
• Green beans give a boost of fiber with relatively few calories, keeping you feeling full longer.

MASHED SWEET POTATOES WITH BROWN SUGAR AND ORANGE

SERVES 4

*I*f you like sweet potatoes, you'll love the simple but intensely flavored additions in this dish. It's another step toward exploring new taste combinations with your reawakened taste buds. Serve with Sunday Roast Chicken (page 214) and a crisp green salad.

2 medium sweet potatoes (about
   1½ pounds)
½ cup (firmly packed) dark
   brown sugar

½ cup fresh orange juice, plus
   extra if needed
½ teaspoon salt

1. Preheat the oven to 425°F. On a baking sheet, bake the potatoes for 60 to 70 minutes, until very tender when pierced with a fork.

2. Remove the potatoes from the oven, maintaining the oven temperature, and place them in an ovenproof bowl or serving dish. When cool enough to handle, peel the potatoes and add the brown sugar, ½ cup orange juice, and salt.

3. Mash the potato mixture with a masher or hand mixer until smooth. Add more orange juice if necessary to reach the desired consistency. Return to the oven to reheat if necessary, and serve hot.

Per Serving: calories, 260; fat (g), 0; carbohydrates (g), 62; protein (g), 3; cholesterol (mg), 0; sodium (mg), 300.

HEALTH CHECK

• Sweet potatoes are an excellent source of beta carotene, an antioxidant that protects against developing cancer, for which smokers are at increased risk.

• When you crave a high-carbohydrate food, your body may need the serotonin that was previously supplied by nicotine. The starch in sweet potatoes will help raise the serotonin level in your brain and calm you down.

• Orange juice adds a shot of vitamin C, which is generally lacking in smokers' diets. Vitamin C is an antioxidant that may help to destroy the process that forms cancer cells.

VEGETABLE MARINADE

MAKES ½ CUP

*T*his is my favorite marinade for grilled vegetables. I use an oiled grill topper and place it on my barbecue to avoid losing any of the delicious vegetables to the fire.

3 tablespoons red wine vinegar

2 tablespoons dry wine or sherry

2 tablespoons sugar or equivalent amount of sugar substitute

1 tablespoon Tabasco sauce

1 tablespoon low-sodium soy sauce

1 tablespoon sesame oil

1 tablespoon chopped garlic

Vegetables of your choice, such as sliced zucchini, yellow squash, green onions (scallions), eggplant, bell peppers (red, yellow, and green), and fennel

1. In a Ziploc bag, combine the vinegar, wine, sugar, Tabasco, soy sauce, sesame oil, and garlic.

2. Place any vegetables you wish to marinate in the bag, seal, and shake to coat. Refrigerate for at least 1 hour to overnight. Drain the vegetables and grill or cook as desired.

Per Serving (1 tablespoon marinade, without vegetables): calories, 35; fat (g), 2; carbohydrates (g), 5; protein (g), 0; cholesterol (mg), 0; sodium (mg), 75.

HEALTH CHECK

• An aromatic mix of tangy ingredients adds loads of flavor to vegetables with very little fat.

• Vinegar and Tabasco sauce add a nice zip for new ex-smokers whose taste buds are just waking up.

• Crisp-tender grilled vegetables provide a crunch that soothes the need for oral gratification.

SAUTÉED ZUCCHINI WITH GARLIC
SERVES 2

One of my favorite Italian restaurants brings this delicious zucchini to the table as an appetizer—a low-calorie alternative to the bread that's so easy to munch on while you're waiting for dinner. Now I make it at home as a starter or side dish. The zucchini is cooked in batches to keep the pan hot enough for browning, which is important to achieve the great flavor.

2 teaspoons olive oil	2 medium zucchini, thinly sliced
2 cloves garlic, minced	Salt and black pepper to taste

1. In a large nonstick skillet, heat half the olive oil over medium-high heat. Add half the garlic and cook for about 1 minute, or until fragrant. Be very careful that the garlic does not burn!

2. Add half the zucchini to the pan and cook for about 4 minutes, or until the zucchini and garlic start to brown, stirring often. If the garlic threatens to burn, reduce the heat a little.

3. Transfer the cooked zucchini to a plate and repeat the process with the remaining oil, garlic, and zucchini. Season with salt and pepper and serve immediately.

Per Serving: calories, 65; fat (g), 5; carbohydrates (g), 5; protein (g), 2; cholesterol (mg), 0; sodium (mg), 140.

HEALTH CHECK
- This recipe has only 65 calories per serving.
- Fresh vegetables give a boost of fiber, which fills you up quickly and keeps you feeling full longer.
- Garlic lends a nice zip for new ex-smokers whose taste buds are just waking up.

CHAPTER 19
Desserts

If you think skipping dessert is the secret to avoiding weight gain or losing weight once you've stopped smoking, think again. Many nutrition experts contend that saying no to sweets only makes people more likely to plunder them later. And new research shows that eating a small amount of sugar may help decrease nicotine cravings (see page 45).

Here you'll find some terrific guilt-free desserts. For the chocolate lover, try Chewy Brownies (page 266), Chocolate Birthday Cake (page 268), or Chocolate Pudding (page 269)—all made with lighter ingredients than the traditional versions. For surprisingly delicious fruit desserts, enjoy Baked Oranges (page 264) or Baked Apples with Marsala and Brown Sugar (page 262), Frozen Banana "Ice Cream" (page 265), or Easy Frozen Strawberry-Banana Pie (page 275). To replace the oral satisfaction you once got from lighting and smoking a cigarette, try the Melon Popsicles (page 271). Savor these luscious confections slowly. They'll provide a nice reward for the great task you've undertaken, yet still fit into your day's calorie and fat goals.

BAKED APPLES WITH MARSALA AND BROWN SUGAR

SERVES 2

*T*here's nothing simpler or more comforting than a baked apple for an afternoon or bedtime snack. There are a few secrets to be aware of, however. First, be sure to peel a strip from around the top of each apple. If you don't, the skin will crack and slip as it swells during baking. Also, don't let the pan liquid cook dry and scorch, which will ruin the flavor of the sauce. Pears can be baked in the same manner.

2 large cooking apples, such as Granny Smith, Jonagold, or Rome Beauty

2 teaspoons granulated sugar

2 teaspoons (packed) brown sugar

¼ cup Marsala or rum (or sub-stitute fresh lemon juice or apple juice), plus more if needed

½ teaspoon fresh lemon juice

Low-fat yogurt or low-fat vanilla ice cream (optional)

1. Preheat the oven to 375°F. Using a small paring knife, core each apple to within ½ inch of the bottom, making sure not to cut all the way through so the apple can hold the flavorings. Remove a thin band of peel from around the top of each apple. Place the apples in a small glass or ceramic baking dish just large enough to hold them.

2. In a cup, mix the granulated and brown sugars. Spoon a liberal amount of the mixture in the center of each apple. Sprinkle some of the mixture over the tops of the apples and into the baking dish as well.

3. Pour the ¼ cup Marsala and the lemon juice over the apples and into the pan around the apples. Cover with aluminum foil and bake for about 30 minutes, or until the apples are almost tender. Check occasionally and add more liquid if necessary to keep the pan moist.

4. Remove the foil and bake for 10 to 15 minutes more. The apples should be quite tender but still hold their shape. Remove from the oven, tilt the pan, and spoon any pan liquid over the apples. Serve immediately, with a dollop of low-fat yogurt or vanilla ice cream, if desired.

Per Serving: calories, 170; fat (g), less than 1 g; carbohydrates (g), 40; protein (g), 0; cholesterol (mg), 0; sodium (mg), less than 5 mg.

HEALTH CHECK
• Each serving has less than 1 gram of fat.
• When you quit smoking, you may have more insulin circulating in your blood, which may increase your craving for sweets. This easy-to-make treat helps solve the problem without a calorie overload.
• Fresh fruit gives a boost of fiber with relatively few calories, and thus keeps you feeling full longer. It's a great alternative when you're tempted to reach for a cigarette.

BAKED ORANGES

SERVES 4

*T*his works best with large, thick-skinned navel oranges, and is particularly good prepared in the winter when oranges are at their peak of sweetness. I've also found that crème de menthe makes an unusual but surprisingly delicious flavor combination with the oranges. Experiment with your favorite liqueur, or try sweet Marsala wine.

4 large seedless navel oranges	**4 tablespoons amaretto liqueur, crème de menthe, or Marsala**

1. Preheat the oven to 350°F. Using a small paring knife, cut the core out of each orange, making sure not to cut all the way through the bottom so the orange can hold the liquid. The hole in the top of the orange should be large enough to insert a dessert spoon. Place the oranges in a small glass or ceramic baking dish just large enough to hold them.
2. Drizzle 1 tablespoon of amaretto inside each orange and cover the pan with aluminum foil. Bake for 1 hour, or until the flesh can be scooped out easily with a spoon. Cool slightly before serving.

Per Serving: calories, 120; fat (g), 0; carbohydrates (g), 23; protein (g), 2; cholesterol (mg), 0; sodium (mg), less than 5 mg.

HEALTH CHECK
- This is a fat-free and delicious dessert.
- Oranges add a shot of vitamin C, which is generally lacking in smokers' diets. This antioxidant helps to destroy the process that creates cancer cells.
- Fruit gives a boost of fiber, which contributes to a long-lasting feeling of fullness.

FROZEN BANANA "ICE CREAM"

SERVES 4

*F*inally—a recipe that takes advantage of those overripe bananas that you usually throw out. Keep them in a Ziploc bag in the freezer until you have enough to make a batch of this cool and creamy treat. You can add a few strawberries or raspberries to the food processor for flavor and color variation.

4 ripe bananas, sliced **1 teaspoon vanilla extract**

1. Freeze the banana slices for at least several hours.
2. In a food processor or blender, combine the frozen bananas and vanilla and puree until smooth. Divide among dessert bowls and serve immediately.

Per Serving (½ cup): calories, 110; fat (g), less than 1 g; carbohydrates (g), 27; protein (g), 1; cholesterol (mg), 0; sodium (mg), 0.

HEALTH CHECK
• This recipe has only 110 calories per serving.
• Bananas are a good source of vitamin B_6, which is generally lacking in smokers' diets.
• This frozen banana puree provides a cool, soothing feeling in the back of the throat and calms the nerves during the tough times.

CHEWY BROWNIES

MAKES 16 BROWNIES

*I*f chocolate is what you want, try these luscious, low-fat sweet treats. After many experiments to produce a tempting "diet" brownie, using prune puree and date puree to replace the fat—which my tasters always unanimously rejected—I finally came up with this winner.

By using egg whites instead of whole eggs, and substituting cocoa powder for part of the chocolate, I have been able to reduce the fat to one-third of that in a regular brownie. The flavor, however, is as satisfying as that of the real thing.

2 squares (2 ounces) unsweetened chocolate
2 tablespoons canola oil
2 teaspoons vanilla extract
1 cup granulated sugar
½ cup all-purpose flour
⅓ cup unsweetened cocoa powder
¼ teaspoon baking powder
⅛ teaspoon salt
3 large egg whites
2 teaspoons confectioners' sugar

1. Preheat the oven to 350°F. Spray an 8-inch square baking pan evenly with vegetable oil spray.
2. In a small glass bowl, combine the chocolate squares and the oil. Microwave on High for about 2 minutes, or until the chocolate is melted, stirring every 45 seconds. (Alternatively, combine the mixture in the top of a double boiler; set it over barely simmering water and stir the ingredients until the chocolate is melted). Then remove from the heat and stir in the vanilla.
3. In a large bowl, combine the granulated sugar, flour, cocoa powder, baking powder, and salt and blend thoroughly. Fold in the melted chocolate mixture and then the egg whites; mix until well blended.

4. Pour the batter into the prepared baking pan. Bake for 25 to 30 minutes, or until a toothpick inserted in the center comes out clean. Transfer to a wire rack to cool. Sprinkle with confectioners' sugar and cut into squares.

Per Serving (1 brownie): calories, 105; fat (g), 4; carbohydrates (g), 18; protein (g), 2; cholesterol (mg), 0; sodium (mg), 35.

HEALTH CHECK
- This recipe has only 4 grams of fat per serving.
- Nicotine and sugar have a similar effect on serotonin activity in the brain. This sweet treat may help reduce your craving for a cigarette without sending your calorie count sky-high.
- Lower-fat cocoa powder replaces some of the chocolate, saving fat and calories.

CHOCOLATE BIRTHDAY CAKE

SERVES 12

*E*veryone deserves a piece of cake on their birthday. This deliciously rich cake is still healthier than its traditional counterpart.

1½ cups all-purpose flour

¼ cup unsweetened cocoa powder

1 teaspoon baking soda

¼ teaspoon salt

¼ cup (½ stick) margarine

1 cup sugar

¾ cup low-fat buttermilk

1 tablespoon vanilla extract

¼ cup semisweet chocolate chips (about 1½ ounces)

1 tablespoon skim milk

Fresh raspberries, for garnish (optional)

1. Preheat the oven to 350°F. Coat a 1½-quart ring mold evenly with vegetable oil spray. In a small bowl, combine the flour, cocoa, baking soda, and salt. Stir with a whisk to mix thoroughly and set aside.

2. In a medium saucepan, melt the margarine over low heat. Remove from the heat and stir in the sugar. Add the buttermilk and stir well.

3. Gradually add the flour mixture to the buttermilk mixture, whisking just until blended. Whisk in the vanilla. Pour the batter into the prepared mold and bake for 35 minutes, or until a small knife inserted into the center comes out clean. Transfer the pan to a wire rack and cool the cake completely. Invert the cooled cake carefully onto a serving platter.

4. In a glass measuring cup, combine the chocolate chips and skim milk. Microwave on High for 20 seconds, or until the chocolate is just melted. Stir well until smooth. Drizzle the mixture evenly over the cake. Garnish with fresh raspberries, if desired.

Per Serving: calories, 185; fat (g), 5; carbohydrates (g), 33; protein (g), 3; cholesterol (mg), 0; sodium (mg), 200.

HEALTH CHECK

• This recipe has only 5 grams of fat per serving.

• Just as nicotine reduces your desire to eat by increasing serotonin levels in the brain, a small amount of this sweet treat can have the same effect.

• Quitting smoking can cause more insulin to circulate in the blood, which may increase your craving for sweets. A low-fat food with a small amount of sugar can help stop the craving without a calorie overload.

CHOCOLATE PUDDING

SERVES 2

*H*omemade is always better than store-bought, especially in this case. Made with fresh milk and cocoa powder, this creamy pudding has plenty of flavor without a lot of fat or fillers. To prevent a skin from forming, press a piece of plastic wrap directly on the surface of the pudding before chilling it.

1 large egg white	1 cup skim milk
⅓ cup unsweetened cocoa powder	¼ cup sugar
	⅛ teaspoon salt
1 tablespoon cornstarch	½ teaspoon vanilla extract

1. In a small bowl, lightly beat the egg white and set aside. In a large bowl, sift together the cocoa and cornstarch. Whisk ½ cup of the milk into the cocoa mixture until completely smooth.
2. In a medium saucepan, combine the remaining milk, the sugar, and salt and mix well. Bring to a boil over high heat, whisking constantly. Remove the pan from the heat.
3. Whisk the cocoa mixture into the hot milk mixture. Bring to a boil over medium-high heat and boil for 2 minutes, whisking constantly.
4. Gradually whisk a few spoonfuls of the hot cocoa mixture into the egg whites, whisking constantly. (Adding the mixture slowly prevents the egg white from cooking.) Whisk the egg-white mixture back into the saucepan and cook over medium-low heat for 2 minutes, whisking constantly. Do not allow the mixture to boil. Remove from the heat.
5. Whisk in the vanilla and blend well. Pour the pudding into small dessert dishes or glasses, cover with plastic wrap, and cool to room temperature. Chill for at least 1 hour before serving.

Per Serving: calories, 200; fat (g), 2; carbohydrates (g), 43; protein (g), 9; cholesterol (mg), 2; sodium (mg), 230.

HEALTH CHECK
- Just as nicotine reduces your desire to eat by increasing serotonin levels in the brain, a small amount of this sweet treat can have the same effect.
- Replacing whole milk with skim milk reduces fat.
- Low-fat cocoa powder replaces chocolate, reducing fat and calories substantially.

ICED MOCHA LATTE

SERVES 1

*T*his recipe is a great way to use up the morning's leftover coffee. If you're at home on a warm afternoon and hankering for a sweet, let this simple concoction satisfy and cool.

1 tablespoon Hershey's chocolate syrup

1 tablespoon sugar or equivalent amount of sugar substitute

1 cup hot brewed coffee, regular or decaffeinated

2 cups ice cubes

½ cup nonfat milk

1. In a glass measure or small bowl, combine the chocolate syrup and sugar. Add the hot coffee and stir until thoroughly blended.

2. Place the ice cubes in a tall glass and pour the coffee mixture over them. Top with nonfat milk and serve immediately. If the coffee is very hot, extra ice may be needed.

Per Serving: calories, 140; fat (g), less than .5 g; carbohydrates (g), 31; protein (g), 5; cholesterol (mg), 2; sodium (mg), 90.

HEALTH CHECK

• The sugar in this recipe can help boost the serotonin levels in your brain that were previously raised by nicotine, and thus give you a sense of calm and pleasure.

• Replacing whole milk with skim milk reduces fat.

• This refreshing drink provides a cool, soothing feeling in the back of the throat and calms the nerves during the tough times.

MELON POPSICLES

MAKES 8 POPSICLES OR 28 ICE CUBES

*H*ere's a quick and healthy alternative to store-bought popsicles— they're sure to cool you off on even the hottest summer day. Any kind of melon will work in this recipe, or for even easier fresh fruit pops, fresh orange juice can replace the melon and sugar mixture. Plastic popsicle molds are available where kitchen supplies are sold (Target, Kmart, some supermarkets, etc.).

1 medium very ripe cantaloupe   ½ cup sugar

1. Halve and seed the cantaloupe, then scoop out all the flesh with a large spoon. In a blender or food processor, combine the cantaloupe and sugar and puree the mixture, adding up to ½ cup water as necessary to make a thick liquid.
2. Divide the melon mixture among plastic popsicle molds or 24 ice cube-tray molds. If using popsicle molds, cover and freeze until firm. If using ice cube trays, cover the filled trays with plastic wrap, insert a toothpick into each cube through the plastic, and freeze until firm.
3. Unmold the popsicles by dipping the bottom of the molds or trays into warm water for a few seconds. Serve at once.

Per Serving (1 popsicle or 4 ice cubes): calories, 72; fat (g), 0; carbohydrates (g), 18; protein (g), 0; cholesterol (mg), 0; sodium (mg), 10.

HEALTH CHECK
• One popsicle or 4 melon cubes has less than 80 calories.
• These frozen treats are a great alternative to a cigarette after a meal, and help gratify the urge to put something in the mouth.
• Melon, especially cantaloupe, is high in vitamin A, which is commonly lacking in smokers' diets.

CANTALOUPE WITH YOGURT AND GINGERSNAPS

SERVES 4

*Y*ou won't find a quicker dessert or afternoon snack than this delicious combination of cool melon, creamy yogurt, and crunchy gingersnaps. The tangy lime juice is the perfect foil for the sweet melon.

1 cup nonfat plain yogurt

1 lime

1 cantaloupe, cubed

8 gingersnaps

1. Place the yogurt in a small bowl and set in the center of a decorative serving platter. Halve the lime, then cut 1 thin slice for the garnish.

2. Scatter the cantaloupe around the yogurt, and squeeze the juice of the lime over the cubes. Garnish the yogurt with the reserved slice of lime. Serve with the gingersnaps.

Per Serving: calories, 210; fat (g), 2; carbohydrates (g), 47; protein (g), 6; cholesterol (mg), 1; sodium (mg), 170.

HEALTH CHECK

• Delicious nonfat yogurt replaces heavy cream and saves fat and calories.

• Cantaloupe adds a shot of vitamin C, which is commonly lacking in smokers' diets.

"FORGET-ME-NOT" MERINGUE COOKIES

MAKES 12 TO 15 COOKIES

*M*y friend Sara Jaye grew up in Malibu, California, she and her sister, Hillary, entertained themselves in the kitchen whipping up these easy sweet treats. Little did they know that these melt-in your-mouth cookies were fat-free. They can be left in a turned-off oven overnight, where the heat from the pilot light will dry them out completely, inspiring their name. (If you aren't careful, you might forget they're in the oven!)

4 large egg whites, at room temperature
1 teaspoon vanilla extract

⅛ teaspoon cream of tartar
1 cup sugar

1. Preheat the oven to 225°F. Line a large baking sheet with baking parchment paper. In a large mixing bowl, using an electric mixer, beat the egg whites at medium speed for about 1 minute, or until foamy. Beat in the vanilla and cream of tartar. Increase the speed to high and continue beating while gradually adding the sugar, 1 tablespoon at a time, until the egg whites stand in stiff, glossy peaks.

2. Drop large spoonfuls of the meringue mixture onto the prepared baking sheet, spacing them well apart. Bake for 1 hour, or until meringues are firm and the bottoms are very lightly browned. Cool on the baking sheets, then store in an airtight container. If you have a gas oven and prefer drier meringues, leave the cookies in the oven overnight.

Per Serving (1 cookie): calories, 71; fat (g), 0; carbohydrates (g), 17; protein (g), 1; cholesterol (mg), 0; sodium (mg), 20.

HEALTH CHECK
- These cookies are fat-free.
- The protein in egg whites increases the feeling of fullness, so you eat less and feel full longer.
- When you quit smoking, you may have more insulin circulating in your blood, which may increase your craving for sweets. These cookies offer sugar with very few calories.

CRUNCHY OATMEAL CHOCOLATE CHIP COOKIES

MAKES 4 DOZEN COOKIES

*T*his cookie dough can be refrigerated for up to three days, wrapped tightly in plastic, or frozen for up to four months. That's good news for those who don't trust themselves alone with an entire batch of baked cookies.

½ cup canola oil
½ cup granulated sugar
½ cup (firmly packed) light or dark brown sugar
4 large egg whites or ½ cup liquid egg substitute
1 teaspoon vanilla extract
1½ cups all-purpose flour

1 teaspoon baking powder
¾ teaspoon baking soda
¼ teaspoon salt
1¾ cups old-fashioned oats
1½ cups bran flakes cereal
⅔ cup semisweet chocolate chips (about 4½ ounces)

1. Preheat the oven to 350°F. Coat 2 baking sheets lightly with vegetable oil spray. In a large mixing bowl, using an electric mixer, blend the oil and both sugars at medium speed until light and fluffy. Add the egg whites and vanilla and beat well.

2. In a medium bowl, combine the flour, baking powder, baking soda, and salt and stir together well. Add the flour mixture to the egg mixture and beat at low speed until combined. Stir in the oats, bran flakes, and chocolate chips with a wooden spoon.

3. Drop the dough by level tablespoonfuls onto the prepared baking sheets, spacing them 2 inches apart. Bake for 12 to 14 minutes, or until the cookies are slightly golden. Transfer the cookies to wire racks and cool completely.

Per Serving (1 cookie): calories, 75; fat (g), 3; carbohydrates (g), 10; protein (g), 1; cholesterol (mg), 0; sodium (mg), 55.

HEALTH CHECK
• Nicotine and sugar have a similar effect on serotonin activity in the brain. This sweet treat may help reduce your cravings for a cigarette.
• Egg whites replace whole eggs in this recipe, reducing cholesterol and fat.
• The complex carbohydrates and fiber in oats increase the feeling of fullness, so you eat less and feel full longer.

EASY FROZEN STRAWBERRY-BANANA PIE

SERVES 8

*T*his pie is a snap to make and a definite crowd-pleaser. Be sure to assemble it a few hours before serving so it has time to freeze properly.

3 cups fat-free whipped topping

2 8-ounce cartons nonfat banana or strawberry yogurt

1 9-inch reduced-fat graham cracker pie crust

2 cups fresh strawberries

1 tablespoon sugar

1. In a large bowl, stir together the whipped topping and yogurt until well mixed. Pour the mixture into the pie crust and smooth with the back of a large spoon or rubber spatula. Cover the pie with plastic wrap and place in the freezer for 30 minutes, or until the filling is just firm.

2. While the pie is freezing, hull and thinly slice the strawberries lengthwise. In a medium bowl, toss the strawberries with the sugar and refrigerate until the pie filling is ready.

3. Arrange the strawberry slices in a decorative pattern on the top of the pie, cover again with the plastic wrap, and freeze for about 2 hours more, or until the filling is very firm. Cut into wedges and serve.

Per Serving: calories, 200; fat (g), 3; carbohydrates (g), 34; protein (g), 5; cholesterol (mg), 1; sodium (mg), 160.

HEALTH CHECK
- Each serving has only 3 grams of fat.
- Fat-free whipped topping replaces whipped heavy cream, saving about 20 grams of fat and nearly 200 calories per serving.
- Strawberries provide a shot of vitamin C, which is often lacking in smokers' diets.

Appendix

How to Calculate Your Calorie Need

Following are guidelines for estimates of recommended daily calories, with breakdowns of fat and carbohydrate grams. In each case, a range of values is listed. Choose the lower figure if you're shorter than average, middle-range if you're of average height, and higher figure if you're tall. To determine your calorie need in more detail, see Chapter 5, page 70, and then return to this chart to review the carbohydrate and fat gram ranges. If you need additional help, consult a registered dietitian.

CATEGORY I

(IF YOU WANT TO MAINTAIN WEIGHT; AVOID WEIGHT GAIN)

DAILY ALLOWANCE: 50% CARBOHYDRATE, 25% PROTEIN, 25% FAT

WOMEN	CALORIES	FAT (G)	CARB. (G)	PROTEIN (G)
	1,700–2,000	55 or less	210–250	100–125
	CAL. PER MEAL	FAT PER MEAL	CARB. PER MEAL	PRO. PER MEAL
	400–600	10–20	35–75	25–30
MEN	CALORIES	FAT (G)	CARB. (G)	PROTEIN (G)
	2,400–2,700	75 or less	300–335	150–165
	CAL. PER MEAL	FAT PER MEAL	CARB. PER MEAL	PRO. PER MEAL
	500–850	20–30	60–100	35–55

CATEGORY II

(IF YOU WANT TO LOSE WEIGHT)

DAILY ALLOWANCE: 50% CARBOHYDRATE, 30% PROTEIN, 20% FAT

WOMEN	CALORIES	FAT (G)	CARB. (G)	PROTEIN (G)
	1,500–1,800	30–40	175–225	75–90
	CAL. PER MEAL	FAT PER MEAL	CARB. PER MEAL	PRO. PER MEAL
	300–500	5–10	35–65	15–25

CATEGORY II (cont.)

(IF YOU WANT TO LOSE WEIGHT)

DAILY ALLOWANCE: 50% CARBOHYDRATE, 30% PROTEIN, 20% FAT

MEN	CALORIES	FAT (G)	CARB. (G)	PROTEIN (G)
	1,800–2,200	40–50	300–335	90–110

	CAL. PER MEAL	FAT PER MEAL	CARB. PER MEAL	PRO. PER MEAL
	500–700	5–15	60–85	25–35

Nutritional Value Counter[1]

FOOD	VOL./WEIGHT	CAL.	FAT (G)	CARB. (G)
BEVERAGES				
Beer	12 fl. ounces	147	0	11
Beer, Light	12 fl. ounces	110	0	6.6
Club Soda	12 fl. ounces	0	0	0
Coffee	12 fl. ounces	8	0	0.7
Cola	12 fl. ounces	152	0	38.5
Cola, Diet	12 fl. ounces	0	0	0
Ginger Ale	12 fl. ounces	124	0	31.8
Liquor, 80 Proof	1.5 fl. ounces	97	0	0
Wine	3.5 fl. ounces	72	0	1.4
CANDY & GUM				
Almond Joy	1.7-ounce bar	241	13.1	28.6
Baby Ruth	2.1-ounce bar	289	12.7	39.1
Bubble Yum, Gum	1 piece	25	0	6
Butterfinger	2.16-ounce bar	293	11.4	40
Candy Corn	¼ cup	182	1	44.8
Caramels	5 pieces	170	3	32
Chocolate, Dark	1.45-ounce bar	207	14	24.4
Chocolate, Milk	1.55-ounce bar	226	13.5	26
Chocolate Chips	1 cup	1,351	84.7	178.1
Gum	1 stick	10	0	2.9
Gum, Sugarless	1 stick	5	0	2

FOOD	VOL./WEIGHT	CAL.	FAT (G)	CARB. (G)
CANDY & GUM (cont.)				
Hard Candy	1 ounce	106	0	27.8
Jelly Beans	10 large	103	0.1	26.1
Kit Kat	1.5-ounce bar	219	11.2	26.7
Life Savers	2 pieces	20	0	5
M&M's	1.69-ounce bag	236	10.1	34.2
Marshmallow	1 regular	23	0	5.9
Milky Way	2.15-ounce bar	258	9.8	43.7
Reese's Peanut Butter Cups	2 pieces	270	15.6	27.3
Three Musketeers	2.13-ounce bar	250	7.7	46.1
CEREALS				
All-Bran, Kellogg's	½ cup	81	1.1	23
Bulgur, Cooked	1 cup	151	0.4	33.8
Cheerios	1 cup	110	2	23
Corn Flakes, Kellogg's	1 cup	102	0.2	24
Cream of Wheat, Cooked	¾ cup	116	0.4	23.7
Farina, cooked	¾ cup	88	0.2	18.6
Froot Loops	1 cup	120	0.9	28.2
Frosted Flakes, Kellogg's	¾ cup	119	0.2	28.4
Granola, Post	⅔ cup	280	9	45
Grape Nuts	½ cup	200	1	47
Malt-O-Meal, cooked	1 cup	100	0.4	21.1
Oats, Quick-Cooking, Uncooked	1 pkg.	104	1.8	18.1
Oats, Old-Fashioned, Uncooked	½ cup	148	3	27.3
Puffed Rice	1 cup	56	0.1	12.6
Raisin Bran, Kellogg's	1 cup	197	1.5	47.1
Rice Krispies	1¼ cups	120	0.2	28.5
Shredded Wheat	1 ounce	102	0.5	23
Total, General Mills	¾ cup	110	1	24
Wheaties	1 cup	110	1	24

FOOD	VOL./WEIGHT	CAL.	FAT (G)	CARB. (G)
CHEESE				
American Processed	1 ounce	106	8.9	0.5
Blue	1 ounce	100	8.1	0.7
Brie	1 ounce	95	7.8	0.1
Cheddar	1 ounce	114	9.4	0.4
Cheddar, Low-Fat	1 ounce	49	2	0.5
Cottage Cheese, 1%	1 cup	164	2.3	6.1
Cottage Cheese, Nonfat	1 cup	160	0	8
Cream Cheese	1 ounce	99	9.9	0.8
Cream Cheese, Light	1 ounce	70	5	2
Feta	1 ounce	75	6	1.2
Monterey Jack	1 ounce	106	8.6	0.2
Mozzarella, Part-Skim	1 ounce	72	4.5	0.8
Parmesan	1 ounce	111	7.3	0.9
Ricotta Part-Skim	½ cup	171	9.8	6.4
Swiss	1 ounce	107	7.8	1
CHIPS AND OTHER SNACKS				
Corn Chips	1 ounce	153	9.5	16.1
Popcorn	3.5 cups	107	1.2	21.8
Potato Chips	1 ounce	152	9.8	15
Pretzels	1 ounce	108	1	22.5
Rice Cake	1 cake	35	0.3	7.5
Tortilla Chips	1 ounce	142	7.4	17.8
DESSERTS				
Angel Food Cake	1 ounce	73	0.2	16.4
Animal Crackers	11 pieces	126	3.9	21
Brownie	(2¾ × ⅞-inch)	227	9.1	35.8
Carrot Cake	½ of 9-inch cake	239	11	32.7
Cheesecake	½ of 9-inch cake	457	33.3	32.3
Chocolate Cake	½ of 9-inch cake	340	14.3	50.7
Chocolate Chip Cookies, Chips Ahoy	3 cookies	160	8	21

FOOD	VOL./WEIGHT	CAL.	FAT (G)	CARB. (G)
DESSERTS (cont.)				
Fig Newtons	2 cookies	110	2.5	20
Frozen Yogurt	½ cup	115	4.3	17.9
Ice Cream, Chocolate	½ cup	143	7.3	18.6
Ice Cream, Vanilla	½ cup	133	7.3	15.6
Jell-O Gelatin	½ cup	83	0	19.6
Oatmeal Cookie	1 cookie	81	3.3	12.4
Peanut Butter Cookie	1 cookie	72	3.5	8.8
Pie, Apple	⅛ of 9-inch pie	411	19.4	57.5
Pie, Cherry	⅛ of 9-inch pie	486	22	69.3
Pie, Lemon Meringue	⅛ of 9-inch pie	362	16.4	49.7
Pie, Peach	⅛ of 9-inch pie	301	12.6	45.1
Pie, Pumpkin	⅛ of 9-inch pie	316	14.4	40.9
Pudding, Chocolate	½ cup	151	2.8	28
Pudding, Vanilla	½ cup	148	2.4	28.1
White Cake	¹⁄₁₂ of 9-inch cake	264	9.2	42.3
EGGS AND EGG SUBSTITUTES				
Egg, Boiled	1 large	78	5.3	0.6
Egg, Fried	1 large	92	6.9	0.6
Egg, Poached	1 large	75	5	0.6
Egg Beaters	¼ cup	30	0	1
Just Whites Powdered Egg Whites	2 teaspoons	14	0	0
Scramblettes Powdered Egg Product	2 tablespoons	35	0	1
FAST FOODS				
Burger King				
Biscuit with Sausage	1 biscuit	590	40	41
Cheeseburger	1 sandwich	380	19	28
Chicken Sandwich	1 sandwich	710	43	54
Fish Sandwich	1 sandwich	700	41	56
French Fries	1 medium serving	370	20	43

FOOD	VOL./WEIGHT	CAL.	FAT (G)	CARB. (G)
Burger King (cont.)				
Hamburger	1 sandwich	330	15	28
Hash Browns	1 serving	220	12	25
Salad, Chicken (no dressing)	1 salad	200	10	7
Salad, Garden (no dressing)	1 salad	100	5	7
Shake, Chocolate	1 medium	320	7	54
Shake, Vanilla	1 medium	300	6	53
Whopper	1 sandwich	640	39	45
Whopper with Cheese	1 sandwich	730	46	46
Hardee's				
Bacon & Egg Biscuit	1 sandwich	570	33	45
Big Country Breakfast with Sausage	1 breakfast	1,000	66	62
Boss Burger	1 sandwich	570	33	42
Cheeseburger	1 sandwich	310	14	30
Chicken Fillet Sandwich	1 sandwich	480	18	54
Cone, Chocolate	1 cone	180	2	34
Cone, Vanilla	1 cone	170	2	34
Fisherman's Fillet	1 sandwich	560	27	54
French Fries	1 large serving	430	18	58
Fried Chicken, Breast	1 piece	370	15	29
Grilled Chicken Salad (no dressing)	1 salad	150	3	11
Roast Beef Sandwich	1 sandwich	320	18	26
Shake, Chocolate	1 shake	370	5	67
Shake, Strawberry	1 shake	420	4	83
Shake, Vanilla	1 shake	350	5	65
Sundae, Hot Fudge	1 sundae	290	6	51
Jack in the Box				
Breakfast Jack	1 sandwich	300	12	30
Cheeseburger, Ultimate	1 sandwich	1,030	79	30
Cheesecake	1 serving	310	18	29

FOOD	VOL./WEIGHT	CAL.	FAT (G)	CARB. (G)
Jack in the Box (cont.)				
Chicken Sandwich, Spicy Crispy	1 sandwich	560	27	55
Chicken Strips	4 pieces	290	13	18
Chicken Teriyaki Bowl	1 bowl	580	1.5	115
Curly Fries, Seasoned	1 serving	360	20	39
Egg Rolls	3 pieces	440	24	54
French Fries	1 medium serving	350	17	45
Garden Chicken Salad (no dressing)	1 salad	200	9	8
Grilled Sourdough Burger	1 sandwich	670	43	39
Jumbo Jack	1 sandwich	560	32	41
Onion Rings	1 serving	380	23	38
Shake, Chocolate	1 shake	630	27	85
Shake, Strawberry	1 shake	640	28	85
Shake, Vanilla	1 shake	610	31	73
Taco	1 taco	190	11	15
Kentucky Fried Chicken				
Biscuit	2-ounce biscuit	180	10	20
Colonel's Crispy Strips	3 strips	261	15.8	10
Cornbread	2-ounce piece	228	13	25
Extra Tasty Crispy Chicken Breast	5.9 ounces	470	28	25
Extra Tasty Crispy Chicken Thigh	4.2 ounces	370	25	18
Green Beans	4.7 ounces	45	1.5	7
Hot & Spicy Breast	6.5 ounces	530	35	23
Hot & Spicy Thigh	3.8 ounces	370	27	13
Macaroni & Cheese	5.4 ounces	180	8	21
Mashed Potatoes with Gravy	4.8 ounces	120	6	17
Original Recipe Breast	5.4 ounces	400	24	16
Original Recipe Thigh	3.2 ounces	250	18	6
Tender Roast Breast	4.9 ounces	251	10.8	1
Tender Roast Thigh	3.2 ounces	207	12	0

FOOD	VOL./WEIGHT	CAL.	FAT (G)	CARB. (G)
McDonald's				
Apple Pie	1 pie	260	14.8	30
Big Mac	1 sandwich	560	32.4	42.5
Biscuit with Sausage & Egg	1 sandwich	520	34.5	32.6
Cheeseburger	1 sandwich	310	13.8	31.2
Chicken McNuggets	1 serving	290	16.3	16.5
Chunky Chicken Salad (no dressing)	1 salad	140	3.4	5.3
Egg McMuffin	1 sandwich	290	11.2	28.1
Fillet-O-Fish	1 sandwich	440	26.1	37.9
French Fries	1 medium serving	320	17.1	36.3
Hamburger	1 sandwich	260	9.5	30.6
Hash Browns	1 serving	130	7.3	14.9
Hot Caramel Sundae	1 sundae	270	2.8	59.3
Quarter Pounder	1 sandwich	410	20.7	34
Pizza Hut				
Bigfoot Pizza, Cheese	1 slice	186	6	25
Hand-Tossed Pizza, Pepperoni	3.7-ounce slice	238	8	29
Hand-Tossed Pizza, Supreme	4.8-ounce slice	284	12	30
Pan Pizza, Meat Lover's	4.6-ounce slice	340	18	28
Pan Pizza, Veggie Lover's	4.8-ounce slice	243	10	29
Personal Pan Pizza, Pepperoni	9-ounce pizza	637	28	69
Thin 'N' Crispy, Cheese	3-ounce slice	205	8	21
Thin 'N' Crispy, Ham	3-ounce slice	184	7	21
Taco Bell				
Bean Burrito	1 burrito	373	12	54.6
Burrito Supreme	1 burrito	449	18.4	50.2
Fajita, Chicken	1 fajita	461	21.2	49.3
Fajita, Steak	1 fajita	465	21.3	47.7
Nachos Bell Grande	1 serving	774	38.8	83.2
Salsa	1 serving	24	0	5
Soft Taco	1 taco	226	9.7	20
Taco	1 taco	183	9.7	11.1
Taco Salad with Salsa	1 salad	431	21.5	29.3

FOOD	VOL./WEIGHT	CAL.	FAT (G)	CARB. (G)
Wendy's				
Cheeseburger	4.1-ounce sandwich	320	10	34
Chicken Club Sandwich	7.6-ounce sandwich	470	20	44
Chili, Large	12-ounce serving	310	10	32
Deluxe Garden Salad	1 salad	110	6	10
French Fries	1 medium serving	380	19	47
Hamburger	4.7-ounce sandwich	360	16	31
Potato, Baked with Bacon & Cheese	1 potato	540	18	78
Stuffed Pita, Chicken Caesar	8.4-ounce sandwich	490	17	46
Taco Salad	1 salad	590	30	53

FATS, OILS, AND SHORTENINGS

FOOD	VOL./WEIGHT	CAL.	FAT (G)	CARB. (G)
Canola Oil	1 tablespoon	124	14	0
Coconut Oil	1 tablespoon	121	14	0
Cod Liver Oil	1 tablespoon	126	14	0
Corn Oil	1 tablespoon	124	14	0
Crisco Shortening	1 tablespoon	110	12	0
Olive Oil	1 tablespoon	124	14	0
Peanut Oil	1 tablespoon	124	14	0
Vegetable Oil Spray	1 spray	2	0.2	0

FISH AND SHELLFISH

FOOD	VOL./WEIGHT	CAL.	FAT (G)	CARB. (G)
Anchovy, Canned	5 anchovies	42	1.9	0
Bass, Raw	3 ounces	97	3.1	0
Catfish, Raw	3 ounces	115	6.5	0
Caviar, Black or Red	1 tablespoon	40	2.9	0.6
Clams, Raw	3 ounces	63	0.8	2.2
Cod, Raw, Atlantic	3 ounces	70	0.6	0
Crab, Raw, Alaskan	3 ounces	71	0.5	0
Crayfish, Raw	3 ounces	65	0.8	0
Halibut, Raw	3 ounces	134	7.7	0
Lobster, Raw	3 ounces	77	0.8	0.4
Mackerel, Raw	3 ounces	174	11.8	0

FOOD	VOL./WEIGHT	CAL.	FAT (G)	CARB. (G)
FISH AND SHELLFISH (cont.)				
Mussels, Raw	3 ounces	73	1.9	3.1
Orange Roughy, Raw	3 ounces	59	0.6	0
Oysters, Raw	6 medium	50	1.3	4.6
Salmon, Raw, Atlantic	3 ounces	156	9.2	0
Salmon, Raw, Pink	3 ounces	99	2.9	0
Scallops, Raw, Bay	3.5 ounces	88	1	2.9
Shrimp, Raw	3 ounces	90	1.5	0.8
Swordfish, Raw	3 ounces	103	3.4	0
Trout, Raw, Rainbow	3 ounces	117	4.6	0
Tuna, Raw, Bluefin	3 ounces	122	4.2	0
Tuna, Canned in Water, White	3 ounces	109	2.5	0
Yellowtail, Raw	3 ounces	124	4.5	0
FRUIT AND VEGETABLE JUICES				
Apple Juice	8 fl. ounces	117	0.3	29
Carrot Juice	6 fl. ounces	74	0.3	17.1
Grape Juice	8 fl. ounces	154	0.2	37.8
Grapefruit Juice	8 fl. ounces	96	0.2	22.7
Lemon Juice	1 tablespoon	4	0	1.3
Lime Juice	1 tablespoon	4	0	1.4
Orange Juice	8 fl. ounces	112	0.5	25.8
Pineapple Juice	8 fl. ounces	130	0.1	31.9
Prune Juice	8 fl. ounces	182	0.1	44.7
Tomato Juice	6 fl. ounces	31	0.1	7.7
V-8 Juice	8 fl. ounces	50	0	10
FRUITS				
Apple	1 medium	81	0.5	21
Applesauce, Unsweetened	½ cup	52	0.1	13.8
Apricots, Dried	10 halves	83	0.2	21.6
Apricots, Fresh	3 medium	51	0.4	11.8
Avocado	1 medium	306	30	12
Banana	1 medium	105	0.5	26.7

FOOD	VOL./WEIGHT	CAL.	FAT (G)	CARB. (G)
FRUIT (cont.)				
Blackberries	½ cup	37	0.3	9.2
Blueberries	1 cup	81	0.6	20.5
Cantaloupe	1 cup chunks	56	0.4	13.4
Cherries	10 cherries	49	0.7	11.3
Dates, Dried	10 dates	228	0.4	61
Fig	1 medium	37	0.1	9.6
Grapefruit	½ medium	39	0.1	9.9
Grapes	1 cup	58	0.3	15.8
Kiwi	1 medium	46	0.3	11.3
Lemon	1 medium	17	0.2	5.4
Mango	1 medium	135	0.6	35.2
Nectarine	1 medium	67	0.6	16
Orange, Navel	1 medium	60	0.1	15.2
Peach	1 medium	37	0.1	9.7
Pear	1 medium	98	0.7	25.1
Pineapple, Raw	1 cup chunks	76	0.7	19.2
Plum	1 medium	36	0.4	8.6
Prunes, dried	10 prunes	201	0.4	52.7
Raisins, seedless	⅔ cup	300	0.5	79.1
Raspberries	1 cup	60	0.7	14.2
Strawberries	1 cup	45	0.6	10.5
Tangerine	1 medium	37	0.2	9.4
Watermelon	1 cup chunks	51	0.7	11.5
GRAIN PRODUCTS				
Bagel, egg	1 bagel (3½ in.)	197	1.5	37.6
Bagel, plain	1 bagel (3½ in.)	195	1.1	37.9
Biscuit, plain	1 biscuit (2½ in.)	127	5.8	17
Cornbread, from mix (3¾ × 2½-inch)	1 slice	188	6	28.9
Blueberry Muffin	1 muffin (2½ in.)	158	3.7	27.4
Bran'ola Bread	1 slice	90	2	18
Brown Rice, cooked	1 cup	216	1.8	44.8
English Muffin	1 muffin	134	1	26.2
French Bread	1 slice	81	1.1	14.8

FOOD	VOL./WEIGHT	CAL.	FAT (G)	CARB. (G)
GRAIN PRODUCTS (cont.)				
Hamburger/Hot Dog	1 bun	123	2.2	21.6
Honey Wheat Berry	1 slice	90	1.5	19
Italian Bread	1 slice	81	1.1	15
Kaiser Roll	1 roll	140	3.5	25
Pancake, From Mix	4-inch cake	74	0.9	13.9
Pasta, Egg, Cooked	2 ounces	74	1	13.3
Pasta, Macaroni, Cooked	1 cup	197	0.9	39.7
Pasta, Spaghetti, Cooked	1 cup	197	0.9	39.7
Pita Bread	1 pita (6½ in. dia.)	165	0.7	33.4
Pumpernickel	1 slice	80	1	15.2
Rye	1 slice	83	1.1	15.5
Sourdough	1 slice	93	0.8	20.7
Tortilla, Corn	1 medium	56	0.6	11.7
Tortilla, Flour	1 7–8 in. tortilla	114	2.5	19.5
Waffle, From Mix	1 7-inch waffle	218	10.3	26.4
Wheat, Bran'ola	1 slice	90	2	16
White Bread	1 slice	67	0.9	12.4
White Rice, Cooked	1 cup	205	0.4	44.5
Wild Rice, Cooked	1 cup	166	0.6	35
MEATS				
Beef				
Brisket, Braised, Trimmed	3.5 ounces	291	19.5	0
Chuck Roast, Braised, Trimmed	3.5 ounces	260	14.6	0
Flank, Braised, Trimmed	3.5 ounces	263	16.4	0
Ground, Extra-Lean, Well-Broiled	3.5 ounces	265	15.8	0
Ground, Regular, Well-Broiled	3.5 ounces	292	19.5	0
Ribs, Broiled, Trimmed	3.5 ounces	237	13.8	0
Round, Bottom, Braised, Trimmed	3.5 ounces	213	8.7	0

FOOD	VOL./WEIGHT	CAL.	FAT (G)	CARB. (G)
Beef (cont.)				
Round, Top, Braised, Trimmed	3.5 ounces	207	5.8	0
Tenderloin, Broiled, Trimmed	3.5 ounces	212	10.1	0
Top Sirloin, Broiled, Trimmed	3.5 ounces	200	7.8	0
Lamb				
Leg, Domestic, Roasted, Trimmed	3.5 ounces	180	6.7	0
Pork				
Bacon, Pan-Fried	3 med. slices	109	9.4	0.1
Center Loin, Braised, Trimmed	3.5 ounces	202	8.3	0
Ham, Cured, Lean	3.5 ounces	145	5.5	1.5
Loin Blade, Braised, Trimmed	3.5 ounces	225	13.1	0
Loin, Braised, Trimmed	3.5 ounces	204	9.1	0
Sausage, Fresh, Cooked	1 link, 1.5 ounces	48	4.1	0.1
Meats, Luncheon				
Bologna, Beef	1-ounce slice	72	6.6	0.2
Bologna, Turkey	1-ounce slice	56	4.3	0.3
Chicken Breast, oven-roasted	1-ounce slice	28	5.1	0.6
Frankfurter, Beef	2-ounce frank	180	16.2	1
Frankfurter, Turkey	2-ounce frank	102	8	0.7
Ham, Sliced, Lean	1-ounce slice	37	1.4	0.3
Salami, Beef	½-ounce slice	60	4.8	0.6
Salami, Pork	⅓-ounce slice	41	3.4	0.2
Turkey Breast	1-ounce slice	29	0.3	0.6
Turkey Pastrami	1-ounce slice	31	0.2	1.1
Veal				
Loin, Braised, Trimmed	3.5 ounces	226	9.2	0

FOOD	VOL./WEIGHT	CAL.	FAT (G)	CARB. (G)
MILK AND YOGURT				
Buttermilk	8 fl. ounces	99	2.2	11.7
Chocolate Milk, 2%	8 fl. ounces	179	5	26
Condensed Milk, Sweetened	1 fl. ounce	122	3.3	20.7
Evaporated Milk, Low-Fat	1 fl. ounce	25	0.5	3
Low-fat Milk, 1%	8 fl. ounces	102	2.6	11.7
Low-fat Milk, 2%	8 fl. ounces	121	4.7	11.7
Nonfat Milk	8 fl. ounces	86	0.4	11.9
Soy Milk	8 fl. ounces	79	4.6	4.3
Whole Milk	8 fl. ounces	150	8.1	11.4
Low-fat Yogurt, 1%	8 fl. ounces	225	2.6	42.3
Nonfat Yogurt	8 fl. ounces	127	0.4	17.4
Whole Yogurt	8 fl. ounces	139	7.4	10.6
NUTS AND SEEDS				
Almonds, Blanched	1 ounce	174	14.4	5.2
Cashews, Roasted	1 ounce	163	13.1	9.3
Chestnuts, Roasted	1 ounce	69	0.6	15
Corn Nuts	1 ounce	124	4	20.8
Macadamias	1 ounce	199	20.9	3.9
Peanut Butter, Chunky	2 tablespoons	188	16	6.9
Peanut Butter, Creamy	2 tablespoons	190	16.3	6.2
Peanuts, Roasted	1 ounce	166	14.1	6.1
Pecans, Roasted	1 ounce	187	18.3	6.3
Pine Nuts	1 ounce	160	14.4	4
Pistachios, Roasted	1 ounce	172	15	7.8
Pumpkin Seeds, Roasted	1 ounce	148	11.9	3.8
Sesame Seeds	1 tablespoon	47	4.4	0.8
Sunflower Seeds, Roasted	1 ounce	165	14.1	6.8
Walnuts	1 ounce	172	16	3.4

FOOD	VOL./WEIGHT	CAL.	FAT (G)	CARB. (G)
POULTRY				
Chicken				
Dark (without skin), Roasted	3.5 ounces	205	9.7	0
Dark (with skin), Roasted	3.5 ounces	253	15.8	0
Light (without skin), Roasted	3.5 ounces	173	4.5	0
Light (with skin), Roasted	3.5 ounces	222	10.8	0
Turkey				
Dark (without skin), Roasted	3.5 ounces	187	7.2	0
Dark (with skin), Roasted	3.5 ounces	221	11.5	0
Light (without skin), Roasted	3.5 ounces	157	3.2	0
Light (with skin), Roasted	3.5 ounces	197	8.3	0
SOUPS				
Bean with Bacon, Campbell's	½ cup	180	5	25
Beef with Veg & Barley, Campbell's	½ cup	80	2	11
Broccoli, Cream of, Campbell's	½ cup	100	6	9
Chicken Noodle, Campbell's	½ cup	70	2	9
Clam Chowder, Campbell's	½ cup	100	2.5	15
Minestrone, Campbell's	½ cup	70	2.5	11
Mushroom, Cream of, Campbell's	½ cup	110	7	9
Split Pea with Ham, Campbell's	½ cup	180	3.5	28
Tomato, Campbell's	½ cup	100	2	18
Vegetable, Campbell's	½ cup	80	1.5	14
SPREADS				
Butter	1 tablespoon	108	12.2	0
Butter, Whipped	1 tablespoon	79	8.9	0
Margarine, Stick	1 tablespoon	100	11	0
Margarine, Stick, Light	1 tablespoon	50	6	1
Mayonnaise	1 tablespoon	100	11	0.1
Mayonnaise, Light	1 tablespoon	50	5	1

FOOD	VOL./WEIGHT	CAL.	FAT (G)	CARB. (G)
SUGARS, SYRUPS, AND SWEETENERS				
Honey	1 tablespoon	64	0	17.3
Jam and Preserves	1 tablespoon	48	0	12.9
Molasses	1 tablespoon	53	0	13.8
Sugar, Brown	1 tablespoon	52	0	13
Sugar, White, Granulated	1 tablespoon	50	0	13
Sugar, White, Powdered	1 tablespoon	31	0	8
Syrup, Corn, Dark	1 tablespoon	56	0	15.3
Syrup, Pancake, Aunt Jemima	¼ cup	212	0.1	52.6
Syrup, Pancake, Reduced-Calorie, S&W	¼ cup	60	0	15
VEGETABLES AND LEGUMES				
Alfalfa Sprouts	1 cup	10	0.2	1.2
Artichoke, Boiled	1 medium	150	0.5	33.5
Asparagus, Boiled	½ cup	22	0.3	3.8
Beets, Boiled	½ cup slices	37	0.2	8.5
Black Beans, Boiled	1 cup	227	0.9	40.8
Broccoli, Boiled	½ cup	22	0.3	3.9
Brussels Sprouts, Boiled	½ cup	30	0.4	6.8
Cabbage, Raw	¼ cup shredded	9	0.1	1.9
Carrot, Raw	1 medium	31	0.1	7.3
Cauliflower, Boiled	½ cup pieces	14	0.3	2.5
Celery, Raw	1 stalk	6	0.1	1.5
Chickpeas (Garbanzo Beans), Canned	1 cup	286	2.7	54.3
Corn, Boiled	½ cup	89	1	20.6
Eggplant, Raw	½ cup	11	0.1	2.5
Great Northern Beans, Canned	1 cup	299	1	55.1
Green Beans, Boiled	½ cup	22	0.2	4.9
Kidney Beans, Canned	1 cup	207	0.8	38.1
Lentils, cooked	1 cup	230	0.8	39.9
Lettuce, Romaine	½ cup	4	0.1	0.7

FOOD	VOL./WEIGHT	CAL.	FAT (G)	CARB. (G)
VEGETABLES AND LEGUMES (cont.)				
Lima Beans, Cooked	1 cup	216	0.7	39.3
Mushrooms, Raw	½ cup pieces	9	0.1	1.6
Mustard Greens, Cooked	½ cup chopped	11	0.2	1.5
Navy Beans, Canned	1 cup	296	1.1	53.6
Onions, Raw	½ cup chopped	30	0.1	6.9
Peas, Green, Cooked	½ cup	62	0.2	11.4
Peppers, Bell, Raw	½ cup chopped	14	0.1	3.2
Pinto Beans, Canned	1 cup	206	1.9	36.6
Potato, Baked	1 potato	220	0.2	51
Pumpkin, Canned	½ cup	122	0.3	9.9
Soybeans, Boiled	1 cup	298	15.4	17.1
Spinach, Raw	½ cup chopped	6	0.1	1
Squash, Summer, Raw	½ cup slices	12	0.2	2.6
Squash, Zucchini, Raw	½ cup slices	9	0.1	1.9
Squash, Butternut, baked	½ cup cubes	41	0.1	10.7
Sweet Potato, Baked	1 potato	117	0.1	27.7
Tomato, Raw	1 tomato	26	0.4	5.7

Stop-Smoking Resources

INTERNET RESOURCES

AMERICA ON-LINE

Go to Addiction and Recovery Forum (A&R), then select the Stop Smoking Today Online Project (S.S.T.O.P.) site for live chat rooms, articles written by Dr. Linda Hyder Ferry, and helpful information on bulletin boards

BLAIR'S QUITTING SMOKING HOME PAGE

Resource pages with links
http://www.chriscor.com/linkstoa.htm

J. CANNON LINKS

Tobacco Resources Center
http://www.gate.net/~jcannon/links.html

CENTERS FOR DISEASE CONTROL: TOBACCO

http://www.cdc.gov/tobacco

DOC (DOCTORS OUGHT TO CARE)

http://www.kickbutt.org/

FOUNDATION FOR INNOVATIONS IN NICOTINE DEPENDENCE (F.I.N.D.)

http://www.findhelp.com

THE MASTER ANTI-SMOKING PAGE
http://www.autonomy.com/smoke.htm

NICOTINE ANONYMOUS
http://www.nicotine-anonymous.org

NO SMOKE CAFE
http://www.clever.net/chrisco/nosmoke/
For people who want to quit smoking, are thinking about quitting smoking, trying to quit, or have already quit
http://www.corral.net/quitters

QUIT NET
http://www.quitnet.org

AGENCY AND COMMUNITY RESOURCES

AGENCY FOR HEALTH CARE POLICY AND RESEARCH PUBLICATION
Publications Clearinghouse
PO Box 8547
Silver Spring, MD 20907
(800) 358-9295 Phone
(301) 594-2800 Fax
http://www.ahcpr.gov

AMERICAN ACADEMY OF FAMILY PHYSICIANS
8880 Ward Parkway
Kansas City, MO 64114-2797
(800) 274-2237

AMERICAN CANCER SOCIETY
1599 Clifton Road NE
Atlanta, GA 30329
(404) 320-3333; (800) 227-2345 Phone
http://www.cancer.org/tobmenu.html

AMERICAN HEART ASSOCIATION

7272 Greenville Avenue
Dallas, TX 75231-4596
(214) 373-6300; (800) 242-8721; or (888) 999-4210 Phone
(214) 706-1341 Fax
http://www.amhrt.org

AMERICAN LUNG ASSOCIATION

1740 Broadway
New York, NY 10019-4374
(800) 586-4872
http://www.lungusa.org

NATIONAL CANCER INSTITUTE'S CANCER INFORMATION SERVICE

(800) 4 CANCER

NATIONAL INSTITUTES OF HEALTH

National Cancer Institute
Publications Ordering Service
PO Box 24128
Baltimore, MD 21227
(800) 422-6237 Phone
(301) 402-5874 Fax
http://cancernet.nci.nih.gov

NICOTINE ANONYMOUS

PO Box 59177
San Francisco, CA 94159-1777
(415) 750-0328; (800) 642-0666 Phone
Call for schedule of meetings
http://www.rampage.org

NATIONAL CENTER FOR CHRONIC DISEASE PREVENTION AND HEALTH PROMOTION CENTERS FOR DISEASE CONTROL, OFFICE OF SMOKING OR HEALTH

1600 Clifton Road
Rhodes Building, MS K-12
Atlanta, GA 30333
(404) 488-5708

SELF-HELP SMOKING CESSATION PROGRAMS

FREEDOM FROM SMOKING
American Lung Association
Check local agency for scheduling of classes

QUITSMART (CAN BE USED IN GROUP SESSIONS)
Robert Shipley, Ph.D.
PO Box 99016, Duke Station
Durham, NC 27708
(888) 73SMART (737-6278) Phone
(919) 286-6934 Fax
http://www.quitsmart.com

SMOKE ENDERS
Check local directory

SMOKE STOPPERS
Check local directory

BOOKS

7 Steps to a Smoke-Free Life. Edwin B. Fisher, Jr. Ph.D., with Toni L. Goldfarb. New York: John Wiley & Sons, Inc. Endorsed by the A.L.A., 1998.

Quit & Stay Quit: A Personal Program to Stop Smoking. Terry A. Rustin, M.D. Center City, Minnesota: Hazelden, 1994.

The Stop Smoking Workbook: Your Guide to Healthy Quitting. Lori Stevic-Rust, Ph.D. and Anita Maximin, Psy.D. Oakland, California: New Harbinger Publications, Inc., 1996.

MISCELLANEOUS WRITTEN MATERIALS

Agency for Health Care Policy and Research
Smoking Cessation: The Consumer Version
Available in English and Spanish, this is an information booklet to increase consumer knowledge and involvement in health care decision making. To order, call (202) 512-1800.

American Cancer Society
Taking Control discusses 10 things a consumer can do to help reduce the risk of cancer and improve peace of mind. American Cancer Society. 1-800-ACS-2345.

When Smokers Quit describes the changes the body goes through beginning 20 minutes after smoking that last cigarette. From *The Health Benefits of Smoking Cessation.* Centers for Disease Control and Prevention DHHS Publication No. (CDC) 90-8416, 1990. Ask for the Stop Smoking Kit E-10-1M.

American Heart Association
(800) 242-8721
Smoking and Heart Disease describes the link between cigarette smoking and major heart and blood vessel disease. Order No. 51-1057, June 1995.

American Lung Association
Facts about . . . Cigarette Smoking
Facts about . . . Is There a Safe Tobacco?
Facts about . . . Nicotine Addiction and Cigarettes
Questions and Answers about Smoking and Health
Quit Smoking Action Plan
(800) 586-4872

National Cancer Institute
Clearing the Air: How to Quit Smoking . . . and Quit for Keeps is an all-inclusive
   consumer guide, with tips on fighting temptation. Describes what to
   expect in the day-to-day process of becoming a nonsmoker. NIH Publication No. 95-1647.
Eat 5 Fruits and Vegetables Every Day provides basic visual examples of
   amounts and sources of needed fruits and vegetables. NIH Publication
   No. 97-3201.
Why Do You Smoke? is a guide to quit smoking that covers the reasons people
   smoke with tips on how to satisfy needs without tobacco. NIH Publication
   No. 94-1822, Revised July 1993.

Notes

INTRODUCTION

1. "Cigarette Smoking Among Adults" United States 1995. *Morbidity and Mortality Weekly Report,* December 26, 1997; 46(51):1217–1220.

CHAPTER ONE

1. Kleseges, R. C., Ward, K. D., Ray J. W., et al. "The Prospective Relationships Between Smoking and Weight in a Young, Biracial Cohort: the Coronary Artery Risk Development in Young Adults Study," *Journal of Consulting and Clinical Psychology.* University of Memphis, 1998; 66 (6):987–993.

CHAPTER TWO

1. *Diagnostic and Statistical Manual for Mental Disorders,* Fourth Edition. American Psychiatric Association, 1994; #292.0.
2. Jorenby, D. E., Leishcow, S. J., Nides, M. A., et al. "A Controlled Trial of Sustained-Release Bupropion, a Nicotine Patch, or Both for Smoking Cessation." *New England Journal of Medicine,* 1999; 340:685–691.
3. Pirie, P. L., McBride, C. M., Hellerstedt W., et al. "Smoking Cessation in Women Concerned with Weight." *American Journal of Public Health,* 1992; 82:1238–1243.
4. Hurt, R., Sachs, D., Glover, E., et al. "A Comparison of Sustained-Release Bupropion and Placebo on Smoking Cessation." *New England Journal of Medicine,* 1997; 337:1195–1202.

5. Anda, R. F., Williamson, D. F., Escobedo, L. G., et al. "Depression and The Dynamics of Smoking." *Journal of the American Medical Association,* 1990; 264:1546–49.

6. Hayford, K. E., Patten, C. A., Rummans, T. A., et al. "Efficacy of Bupropion for Smoking Cessation in Smokers with a Former History of Major Depression or Alcoholism." *British Journal of Psychiatry.* 1999; 174:173–178.

CHAPTER THREE

1. Somer, Elizabeth. *Mood and Food, The Complete Guide to Eating Well and Feeling Your Best,* First Edition. New York: Henry Holt & Co., 1995, p. 17.

APPENDIX

1. Boes and Church. *Food Values of Portions Commonly Used,* 17th edition. Philadelphia: J. B. Lippincott-Raven Publishers, 1998.

Index

Agency and community resources, 294–96
allyl sulfides, 63
antioxidants, 60–63
appendix, 276–92
appetite. *See also* eating habits; food cravings
    effect of endorphins on, 44–45
    effect of insulin on, 41–42
    effect of nicotine on, 10–11
    effect of NPY on, 43–44
    effect of serotonin on, 39–41
Appetizers, 166–70
    Artichokes with Dip, 167
    Ham with Melon, 168
    Refried Bean Dip, 169
    Vegetable Dip for Crudités, 170
Apple, Chicken Salad with, 186
Apple, Cucumber, and Cilantro Salad, 184
Apples, Baked, with Marsala and Brown
    Sugar, 262–63
Applesauce, Pork Chops with, 227
Artichokes with Dip, 167
Avocado, Tomato, and Red Onion Salad,
    196

Bagels with Cream Cheese and Salmon, 239
Baked Apples with Marsala and Brown
    Sugar, 262–63
Baked Garlic Fries, 248
Baked Oatmeal, 153
Baked Oranges, 264
Banana, Frozen, "Ice Cream," 265
Banana Breakfast Smoothie, Orange-, 161
Banana Pie, Easy Frozen Strawberry-, 275
Banana Toast, Peanut Butter-, 154
Barbecued Chicken, Chili-Rubbed, 210

Barbecued Chicken Chopped Salad, 185
Basic Green Salad with Vinaigrette, 194
Basil
    Pasta with Pesto, 233
    Soup, Tomato and, 180
BBQ Pork Sandwiches, 240
Bean(s), 291–92. *See also* Green Beans
    Barbecued Chicken Chopped Salad, 185
    and Cheese Burritos, Tex-Mex, 245
    Lean Turkey Chili, 221–22
    Meatless Taco Salad, 195
    Refried, Dip, 169
    Spicy Lentil Soup, 177
    White, Salad, 198–99
Beef, 287–88
    Fajitas, 219
    limiting consumption of, 52–53
    Meatballs, 223
    ordering, at restaurants, 139
    Sloppy Joes, 244
    Stew, Old-Fashioned, 225–26
Beer, Grilled Chicken Breasts with, 211
Best Grilled Swordfish, 202
beta carotene, 60–61
beta glucan, 62
beverages, 277
Birthday Cake, Chocolate, 268–69
blood sugar, 42–43
Blueberry Muffins, Honey-Bran, 160
Bran Blueberry Muffins, Honey-, 160
Bran Muffins, Refrigerator Buttermilk,
    164–65
bread. *See also* Muffins; Tortillas
    low-fat, buying, 147
    ordering, in restaurants, 136

breakfast, 46, 135
Breakfast and brunch dishes, 151–65
    Baked Oatmeal, 153
    Buttermilk Pancakes, 155
    Cranberry-Oatmeal Muffins, 156
    Crunchy Granola, 157
    Egg White Omelet with Green Onion
      and Parmesan, 157
    French Toast, 159
    Honey-Bran Blueberry Muffins, 160
    Orange-Banana Breakfast Shake, 161
    Peanut Butter-Banana Toast, 154
    Ranch-Style Eggs with Tortillas, 162–63
    Refrigerator Buttermilk Bran Muffins,
      164–65
Broccoli with Mock Hollandaise Sauce, 249
Broiled Salmon with Garlic, 203
Brownies, Chewy, 266–67
bupropion hydrochloride (Zyban), 31–33
Burgers, French Onion Turkey, 243
Burritos, Tex-Mex Bean and Cheese, 245
butter, 58, 290
Buttermilk, 289
    Bran Muffins, Refrigerator, 164–65
    Pancakes, 155

Cake, Chocolate Birthday, 268–69
calcium, 61–62
calories
    burning, with exercise, 110
    keeping track of, 72–74
    recommended daily, 70–72, 276–77
candy and gum, 277–78
canola oil, 58, 284
Cantaloupe
    Ham with Melon, 168
    Melon Popsicles, 271
    with Yogurt and Gingersnaps, 272
cardiovascular workouts, 111
Carrots and Zucchini with Sesame and Soy,
    250
Cereal, 278
    Baked Oatmeal, 153
    buying, 147
    Crunchy Granola, 157
Cheese, 279
    Burritos, Tex-Mex Bean and, 245
    Chicken Parmesan with Pasta, 231
    Cream, Bagels with Salmon and, 239
    limiting consumption of, 53–54
    Pizza Margarita, 234–35
    Quesadillas, Easy Ham and, 242

Spinach and Zucchini Lasagna, 236–37
    Veggie Wraps, 246
Chewy Brownies, 266–67
Chicken, 290
    Barbecued, Chopped Salad, 185
    Barbecued, Pizza, 229–30
    Breasts with Beer, Grilled, 211
    Chili-Rubbed Barbecued, 210
    increasing consumption of, 52–53
    Jambalaya, 206
    Kabobs, Smoky, 213
    ordering, in restaurants, 138–39
    Oven-Fried, 212
    with Peas, 209
    Piccata, 207
    "Pot Roast," 208
    Salad, Chinese, 187–88
    Salad Sandwiches, 241
    Salad with Apple, 186
    Stir-Fry, Sweet and Sour, 215–16
    Sunday Roast, 214
    Teriyaki, 217
    in Wine, Weekday, 218
Chili, Lean Turkey, 221–22
Chili-Rubbed Barbecued Chicken, 210
Chinese Chicken Salad, 187–88
Chinese restaurants, 138
Chocolate
    Birthday Cake, 268
    Chewy Brownies, 266–67
    Chip Cookies, Crunchy Oatmeal, 274
    cravings for, 45, 49, 119
    Pudding, 269
Chopped Cucumber-Tomato Salad, 189
Chowder, Corn, 172
cocktail parties, snacking at, 124
community and agency resources, 294–96
condiments, buying, 147
Cookies
    Crunchy Oatmeal Chocolate Chip, 274
    "Forget-Me-Not" Meringue, 273
cooking, timesaving tips for, 149–50
Corn
    Barbecued Chicken Chopped Salad, 185
    Chowder, 172
    Meatless Taco Salad, 195
coronary heart disease, 15
Cranberry-Oatmeal Muffins, 156
cravings, food. See food cravings
cravings, nicotine, 11–12
Cream Cheese and Salmon, Bagels with, 239
Creamy Vegetable Soup, 173

Crudités, Vegetable Dip for, 170
Crunchy Cucumber Slices, 190
Crunchy Granola, 157
Crunchy Oatmeal Chocolate Chip Cookies, 274
Cuban-Style Turkey in Tortillas, 220
Cucumber, Apple, and Cilantro Salad, 184
Cucumber Slices, Crunchy, 190
Cucumber-Tomato Salad, Chopped, 189

Dairy products, 289
    buying, 147
    reduced-fat, 56–57
dehydration, 59
deli meats, 146
Desserts, 261–75
    Baked Apples with Marsala and Brown Sugar, 262–63
    Baked Oranges, 264
    Cantaloupe with Yogurt and Ginger-snaps, 272
    Chewy Brownies, 266–67
    Chocolate Birthday Cake, 268
    Chocolate Pudding, 269
    Crunchy Oatmeal Chocolate Chip Cookies, 274
    Easy Frozen Strawberry-Banana Pie, 275
    "Forget-Me-Not" Meringue Cookies, 273
    Frozen Banana "Ice Cream," 265
    Iced Mocha Latte, 270
    Melon Popsicles, 271
    nutritional values of, 279–80
diabetics, 15
diets, 50–51, 66–67, 102
dining out
    Chinese restaurants, 138
    fast food restaurants, 140–41, 280–84
    Italian restaurants, 137–38
    Menu Plans, 92–97
    Mexican restaurants, 137
    ordering beef, 139
    ordering bread, 136
    ordering breakfast, 135
    ordering chicken, 138–39
    ordering fish, 139
    ordering salad, 135
    ordering sandwiches, 136–37
    ordering soups, 136
    tips for, 106, 131–33
Dip, Artichokes with, 167
Dip, Refried Bean, 169
Dip, Vegetable, for Crudités, 170

dopamine, 20
dressings, salad. *See specific salads*
Dry-Roasted Green Beans with Garlic and Soy Sauce, 251

Easy Frozen Strawberry-Banana Pie, 275
Easy Ham and Cheese Quesadillas, 242
eating habits, 12–13. *See also* overeating
    changing, 14–15, 102
    healthy, rules for, 52–62
    new ex-smokers, rules for, 46–49
    television and, 126
Eggs, 280
    Egg White Omelet with Green Onion and Parmesan, 157
    Ranch-Style, with Tortillas, 162–63
endorphins, 44–45
exercise
    calories burned by, 110
    finding time for, 112–14
    goals for, 101, 109
    importance of, 108–9
    prior to quitting, 109
    types of, 111–12

Fad diets, 50–51, 66–67
Fajitas, Beef, 219
fast food restaurants, 140–41, 280–84
fat cravings, 44, 45, 49
fats, 284
fiber, 57, 62
Fish, 284–85
    Bagels with Cream Cheese and Salmon, 239
    Best Grilled Swordfish, 202
    Broiled Salmon with Garlic, 203
    buying, 146
    Grilled, with Tomato Salsa, 204
    increasing consumption of, 52–53
    ordering, in restaurants, 139
folic acid, 61
Food and Exercise Record, 73–74, 113–14
food cravings
    chocolate, 45, 49, 119
    controlling, 72, 99, 107, 119–20, 120–21
    fat, 44, 45, 49
    sugar, 45, 48–49, 99, 104, 119, 120–21
    trigger foods, 122–23
food serving checklist, 65
food shopping tips, 146–48
foods, unprocessed, 47–48, 121

"Forget-Me-Not" Meringue Cookies, 273
French Onion Soup, 174
French Onion Turkey Burgers, 243
French Toast, 159
Fried Rice, 252
Fries, Baked Garlic, 248
Frozen Banana "Ice Cream," 265
frozen foods, 147
Frozen Strawberry-Banana Pie, Easy, 275
fruit juices, 285
fruits, 285–86. See also specific fruits
    buying, 146
    increasing consumption of, 55–56
"fullness," sensation of, 75–76, 104–5

Galanin, 44
Garlic
    Broiled Salmon with, 203
    Fries, Baked, 248
    and Ginger, Stir-Fried Snow Peas with,
        256
    and Lemon, Shrimp with, 205
    Sautéed Zucchini with, 260
    and Soy Sauce, Dry-Roasted Green Beans
        with, 251
Gazpacho, 175
Ginger, Stir-Fried Snow Peas with Garlic
    and, 256
Gingersnaps, Cantaloupe with Yogurt and,
    272
goal-setting, examples of, 99–107
grain products, 57–58, 147, 286–87
Granola, Crunchy, 157
Grated Vegetable Platter with Vinaigrette,
    191–92
Green Beans
    Dry-Roasted, with Garlic and Soy Sauce,
        251
    Sautéed, with Walnuts and Lemon, 257
    Vinaigrette, 193
Green Salad, Basic, with Vinaigrette, 194
green tea, 63
Greens. See Lettuce; Spinach
Grilled Chicken Breasts with Beer, 211
Grilled Fish with Tomato Salsa, 204
Grilled Swordfish, Best, 202
gum and candy, 277–78
Gumbo, Seafood, 178–79

Ham and Cheese Quesadillas, Easy, 242
Ham with Melon, 168
high blood cholesterol levels, 15

high blood pressure, 15, 63
Hollandaise Sauce, Mock, Broccoli with,
    249
Home-Alone Chicken Soup, 176
Honey-Bran Blueberry Muffins, 160
hunger pangs, 75–76, 104

"Ice Cream," Frozen Banana, 265
Iced Mocha Latte, 270
indoles, 62
insulin, 41–43
Internet resources, 292–94
Italian restaurants, 137–38
Italian-Style Spaghetti Squash, 253

Jambalaya, Chicken, 206

Kabobs, Smoky Chicken, 213

Lasagna, Spinach and Zucchini, 236–37
late night snacking, 125–26
Lean Turkey Chili, 221–22
legumes, 291–92. See also Bean(s)
Lemon, Shrimp with Garlic and, 205
Lemon and Walnuts, Sautéed Green Beans
    with, 257
Lentil Soup, Spicy, 177
Lettuce
    Barbecued Chicken Chopped Salad, 185
    Basic Green Salad with Vinaigrette, 194
    Chinese Chicken Salad, 187–88
    Meatless Taco Salad, 195
lycopene, 63

Main Courses, 201–27
    Beef Fajitas, 219
    Best Grilled Swordfish, 202
    Broiled Salmon with Garlic, 203
    Chicken Jambalaya, 206
    Chicken Piccata, 207
    Chicken "Pot Roast," 208
    Chicken with Peas, 209
    Chili-Rubbed Barbecued Chicken, 210
    Cuban-Style Turkey in Tortillas, 220
    Grilled Chicken Breasts with Beer, 211
    Grilled Fish with Tomato Salsa, 204
    Lean Turkey Chili, 221–22
    Meatballs, 223
    Mustard-Glazed Pork Chops, 224
    Old-Fashioned Beef Stew, 225–26
    Oven-Fried Chicken, 212
    Pork Chops with Applesauce, 227

Shrimp with Garlic and Lemon, 205
Smoky Chicken Kabobs, 213
Sunday Roast Chicken, 214
Sweet and Sour Chicken Stir-Fry, 215–16
Teriyaki Chicken, 217
Weekday Chicken in Wine, 218
margarine, 58, 290
Marinade, Vegetable, 259
Mashed Sweet Potatoes with Brown Sugar
    and Orange, 258
meals, skipping, 52
Meatballs, 223
Meatless Taco Salad, 195
Meats, 287–88. *See also* Beef; Pork
    buying, 146
medications, 30–33
meetings, snacking at, 124
Melons. *See* Cantaloupe
menu planning, 145–50
    quick-fix meal ideas, 148–49
Menu Plans
    for dining out, 92–97
    how to use, 79
    for quitting day, 76–78
    week one, 80–85
    week two, 86–91
Meringue Cookies, "Forget-Me-Not," 273
metabolism, 10–12, 108
Mexican restaurants, 137
milk, 289
mineral supplements, 59–63
Mocha Latte, Iced, 270
Mock Hollandaise Sauce, Broccoli with, 249
motivation, 98–99, 103
Muffins
    Cranberry-Oatmeal, 156
    Honey-Bran Blueberry, 160
    Refrigerator Buttermilk Bran, 164–65
Mustard-Glazed Pork Chops, 224

Nasal spray, 31
negative attitudes, overcoming, 99–107
Nicorette gum, 31
nicotine
    cravings, 11–12
    effect on appetite, 10, 39
    effect on brain chemistry, 20–21
    effect on metabolism, 11
    effect on psychological disorders, 34–35
    patches, 31
    replacements, 30–31, 33
    withdrawal symptoms, 29, 45

Nicotrol inhaler, 31
norepinephrine, 20
NPY, 43–44
nutrition, snacks and, 120
nutritional value counter, 277–92
nuts and seeds, 289

Oatmeal
    Baked, 153
    Chocolate Chip Cookies, Crunchy, 274
    Muffins, Cranberry-, 156
oils, 58, 284
Old-Fashioned Beef Stew, 225–26
olive oil, 58, 284
Omelet, Egg White, with Green Onion and
    Parmesan, 158
Onion, Red, Tomato, and Avocado Salad,
    196
Onion Soup, French, 174
Onion Turkey Burgers, French, 243
oral stimulation, 122
Orange-Banana Breakfast Smoothie, 161
Oranges, Baked, 264
Oven-Fried Chicken, 212
overeating
    controlling, by feeling full, 75–76
    controlling, with slower eating, 104–5
    controlling, with smaller meals, 118–19
    snacks, 121–22
    at social events, 124–25
    when dining out, 106

Pancakes, Buttermilk, 155
Pancakes, Potato, 254
pantry items, buying, 147
Parmesan, Chicken, with Pasta, 231
Pasta
    Chicken Parmesan with, 231
    Home-Alone Chicken Soup, 176
    with Pesto, 233
    Spinach and Zucchini Lasagna, 236–37
    Toss, Fresh Tomato, 232
patches, 31
Peanut Butter-Banana Toast, 154
Peas, Chicken with, 209
Personal Nutrition Management Plan. *See
    also* Menu Plans
    four steps of, 68–76
    guidelines for, 79
    smart snacks for, 127–29
Pesto, Pasta with, 233
Piccata, Chicken, 207

Pie, Easy Frozen Strawberry-Banana, 275
Pizza, Barbecued Chicken, 229–30
Pizza Margarita, 234–35
Popsicles, Melon, 271
Pork, 288
    Chops, Mustard-Glazed, 224
    Chops with Applesauce, 227
    Easy Ham and Cheese Quesadillas, 242
    Ham with Melon, 168
    limiting consumption of, 52–53
    Sandwiches, BBQ, 240
portion sizes
    estimating, 134
    in food serving checklist, 64–65
    at restaurants, 131–33
    for snacks, 122
"Pot Roast," Chicken, 208
Potato(es)
    Baked Garlic Fries, 248
    Pancakes, 254
    Roasted Rosemary, 255
    Salad, Warm, 197
    Sweet, Mashed, with Brown Sugar and
        Orange, 258
poultry, 290. See also Chicken; Turkey
    buying, 146
psychological disorders, 34–35
Pudding, Chocolate, 269

Quesadillas, Easy Ham and Cheese, 242
quick-fix meal ideas, 148–49
quitting
    day one, menu for, 76–78
    effect on body, 11–12, 27–28, 59
    enlisting professional help, 30, 36–37
    exercise prior to, 109
    fear of, 3
    obstacles to, 2–3, 37
    reasons for, analyzing, 17–18
    stress resulting from, 105
quizzes, 17–18, 22–24

Ranch-Style Eggs with Tortillas, 162–63
Refried Bean Dip, 169
Refrigerator Buttermilk Bran Muffins,
    164–65
refrigerator staples, 147
restaurants. See dining out
resveratrol, 63
Rice, Fried, 252
Roasted Rosemary Potatoes, 255
Rosemary Potatoes, Roasted, 255

Salad dressings. See specific salads
Salads, 183–200
    Apple, Cucumber, and Cilantro, 184
    Barbecued Chicken Chopped, 185
    Basic Green, with Vinaigrette, 194
    Chicken, Sandwiches, 241
    Chicken, with Apple, 186
    Chinese Chicken, 187–88
    Chopped Cucumber-Tomato, 189
    Crunchy Cucumber Slices, 190
    Grated Vegetable Platter with Vinai-
        grette, 191–92
    Green Beans Vinaigrette, 193
    Meatless Taco, 195
    ordering, in restaurants, 135
    Tomato, Red Onion, and Avocado, 196
    Warm Potato, 197
    White Bean, 198–99
    Wilted Spinach, 200
Salmon, Broiled, with Garlic, 203
Salmon and Cream Cheese, Bagels with, 239
Salsa, Tomato, Grilled Fish with, 204
Sandwiches and Wraps, 238–46
    Bagels with Cream Cheese and Salmon,
        239
    BBQ Pork Sandwiches, 240
    Chicken Salad Sandwiches, 241
    Easy Ham and Cheese Quesadillas, 242
    French Onion Turkey Burgers, 243
    low-fat choices for, 54–55
    ordering, in restaurants, 136–37
    Sloppy Joes, 244
    Tex-Mex Bean and Cheese Burritos, 245
    Veggie Wraps, 246
Sauce, Mock Hollandaise, Broccoli with, 249
sauces, ready-made, buying, 147
Sautéed Green Beans with Walnuts and
        Lemon, 257
Sautéed Zucchini with Garlic, 260
Seafood Gumbo, 178–79
seeds and nuts, 289
selenium, 61
self-defeating thoughts, 98–107
self-help smoking cessation programs, 296
serotonin, 39–41
Sesame and Soy, Carrots and Zucchini with,
        250
shellfish, 284–85. See also Shrimp
shortcut cooking secrets, 149–50
Shrimp
    with Garlic and Lemon, 205
    Seafood Gumbo, 178–79

Side Dishes, 247–60
   Baked Garlic Fries, 248
   Broccoli with Mock Hollandaise Sauce, 249
   Carrots and Zucchini with Sesame and
      Soy, 250
   Dry-Roasted Green Beans with Garlic
      and Soy Sauce, 251
   Fried Rice, 252
   Italian-Style Spaghetti Squash, 253
   Mashed Sweet Potatoes with Brown
      Sugar and Orange, 258
   Potato Pancakes, 254
   Roasted Rosemary Potatoes, 255
   Sautéed Green Beans with Walnuts and
      Lemon, 257
   Sautéed Zucchini with Garlic, 260
   Stir-Fried Snow Peas with Garlic and
      Ginger, 256
   Vegetable Marinade, 259
Sloppy Joes, 244
smokers
   body fat distribution on, 11
   six types of, 24–27
   statistics on, 1
smoking. See also quitting
   effect on appetite, 10–11
   effect on metabolism, 10–11
   health risks from, 19–20
   reasons for, analyzing, 17–18, 21–27
   statistics on, 19
Smoky Chicken Kabobs, 213
Smoothie, Orange-Banana Breakfast, 161
snacks and snacking, 279
   food choices for, 127–29
   guidelines for, 117
   late night, 125–26
   rules for, 118–23
   and weight gain, 116
Snow Peas, Stir-Fried, with Garlic and Gin-
      ger, 256
social events, overeating at, 124–25
soda pop, 59
sodium, 63
Soups, 171–82
   canned, 290
   Corn Chowder, 172
   Creamy Vegetable, 173
   French Onion, 174
   Gazpacho, 175
   Home-Alone Chicken, 176
   ordering, in restaurants, 136
   Seafood Gumbo, 178–79

Spicy Lentil, 177
Tomato and Basil, 180
Vegetable, 181–82
Soy, Carrots and Zucchini with Sesame and,
   250
Soy Sauce, Dry-Roasted Green Beans with
   Garlic and, 251
Spaghetti Squash, Italian-Style, 253
Spicy Lentil Soup, 177
Spinach and Zucchini Lasagna, 236–37
Spinach Salad, Wilted, 200
sports events, 124–25
spreads, 290
Squash, Spaghetti, Italian-Style, 253
Squash, summer. See Zucchini
steak houses, 139
Stew, Old-Fashioned Beef, 225–26
Stir-Fried Snow Peas with Garlic and Gin-
   ger, 256
Stir-Fry, Sweet and Sour Chicken, 215–16
stop-smoking resources, 293–98
Strawberry-Banana Pie, Easy Frozen, 275
strength training, 111, 114–15
stretching exercises, 111
sugar cravings, 45, 48–49, 99, 104, 119,
   120–21
Sunday Roast Chicken, 214
Sweet and Sour Chicken Stir-Fry, 215–16
Sweet Potatoes, Mashed, with Brown Sugar
   and Orange, 258
sweeteners, 291
Swordfish, Best Grilled, 202

Taco Salad, Meatless, 195
television, eating habits and, 126
Teriyaki Chicken, 217
Tex-Mex Bean and Cheese Burritos, 245
Toast, French, 159
Toast, Peanut Butter-Banana, 154
Tomato
   and Basil Soup, 180
   Pasta Toss, Fresh, 232
   Red Onion, and Avocado Salad, 196
   Salad, Chopped Cucumber-, 189
   Salsa, Grilled Fish with, 204
Tortillas
   Beef Fajitas, 219
   Cuban-Style Turkey in, 220
   Easy Ham and Cheese Quesadillas, 242
   Ranch-Style Eggs with, 162–63
   Tex-Mex Bean and Cheese Burritos, 245
   Veggie Wraps, 246

trigger foods, 122–23
Turkey, 290
    Burgers, French Onion, 243
    Chili, Lean, 221–22
    Cuban-Style, in Tortillas, 220
    Meatballs, 223

U.S.D.A. Food Guide Pyramid, 134

Vegetable(s), 291–92. *See also specific vegetables*
    buying, 146
    Dip for Crudités, 170
    Fried Rice, 252
    Gazpacho, 175
    Grated, Platter with Vinaigrette, 191–92
    increasing consumption of, 55–56
    juices, 285
    Marinade, 259
    Ranch-Style Eggs with Tortillas, 162–63
    Soup, 181–82
    Soup, Creamy, 173
    Veggie Wraps, 246
Veggie Wraps, 246
vending machines, 123
Vinaigrette
    Basic Green Salad with, 194
    Grated Vegetable Platter with, 191–92
    Green Beans, 193
vitamin-mineral supplements, 59–63

Walnuts and Lemon, Sautéed Green Beans with, 257
Warm Potato Salad, 197

water, daily consumption of, 59
Weekday Chicken in Wine, 218
weight gain
    attitudes toward, 100, 101, 103
    eating habits as cause of, 12–13
    health risks from, 15
    minimizing, with medications, 33
    reasons for, 9, 12
    statistics on, 10
    women and, 13–14
weight loss
    calculating calories for, 70–72, 276–77
    exercise required for, 110
    giving up on, 106
    realistic goals for, 69–70
weight training, 111, 114–15
weights, buying, 114–15
White Bean Salad, 198–99
whole grains, 57–58, 147, 286–87
Wilted Spinach Salad, 200
Wine, Weekday Chicken in, 218
women, weight gain and, 13–14
Wraps. *See* Sandwiches and Wraps

Yogurt, 289
    and Gingersnaps, Cantaloupe with, 272

Zucchini
    and Carrots with Sesame and Soy, 250
    Sautéed, with Garlic, 260
    and Spinach Lasagna, 236–37
Zyban, 31–33

Conversion Chart
Equivalent Imperial and Metric Measurements

American cooks use standard containers, the 8-ounce cup and a tablespoon that takes exactly 16 level fillings to fill that cup level. Measuring by cup makes it very difficult to give weight equivalents, as a cup of densely packed butter will weigh considerably more than a cup of flour. The easiest way therefore to deal with cup measurements in recipes is to take the amount by volume rather than by weight. Thus the equation reads:

1 cup = 240 ml = 8 fl. oz.   ½ cup = 120 ml = 4 fl. oz.

It is possible to buy a set of American cup measures in major stores around the world.

In the States, butter is often measured in sticks. One stick is the equivalent of 8 tablespoons. One tablespoon of butter is therefore the equivalent to ½ ounce/15 grams.

LIQUID MEASURES

Fluid Ounces	U.S.	Imperial	Milliliters
	1 teaspoon	1 teaspoon	5
¼	2 teaspoons	1 dessertspoon	10
½	1 tablespoon	1 tablespoon	14
1	2 tablespoons	2 tablespoons	28
2	¼ cup	4 tablespoons	56
4	½ cup		110
5		¼ pint or 1 gill	140
6	¾ cup		170
8	1 cup		225
9			250, ¼ liter
10	1¼ cups	½ pint	280
12	1½ cups		340
15		¾ pint	420
16	2 cups		450
18	2¼ cups		500, ½ liter
20	2½ cups	1 pint	560
24	3 cups		675
25		1¼ pints	700
27	3½ cups		750
30	3¾ cups	1½ pints	840
32	4 cups or 1 quart		900
35		1¾ pints	980
36	4½ cups		1000, 1 liter
40	5 cups	2 pints or 1 quart	1120

SOLID MEASURES

U.S. and Imperial Measures		Metric Measures	
Ounces	Pounds	Grams	Kilos
1		28	
2		56	
3½		100	
4	¼	112	
5		140	
6		168	
8	½	225	
9		250	¼
12	¾	340	
16	1	450	
18		500	½
20	1¼	560	
24	1½	675	
27		750	¾
28	1¾	780	
32	2	900	
36	2¼	1000	1
40	2½	1100	
48	3	1350	
54		1500	1½

OVEN TEMPERATURE EQUIVALENTS

Fahrenheit	Celsius	Gas Mark	Description
225	110	¼	Cool
250	130	½	
275	140	1	Very Slow
300	150	2	
325	170	3	Slow
350	180	4	Moderate
375	190	5	
400	200	6	Moderately Hot
425	220	7	Fairly Hot
450	230	8	Hot
475	240	9	Very Hot
500	250	10	Extremely Hot

Any broiling recipes can be used with the grill of the oven, but beware of high-temperature grills.

Equivalents for Ingredients

all-purpose flour—plain flour
coarse salt—kitchen salt
cornstarch—cornflour
eggplant—aubergine

half and half—12% fat milk
heavy cream—double cream
light cream—single cream
lima beans—broad beans

scallion—spring onion
unbleached flour—strong, white flour
zest—rind
zucchini—courgettes or marrow